EXECUTIVE COACHING FOR NURSE LEADERS

EXECUTIVE COACHING FOR NURSE LEADERS

A PRACTICAL GUIDE

ASHLEY SINGH

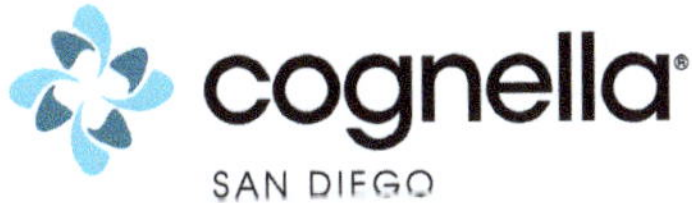

SAN DIEGO

Bassim Hamadeh, CEO and Publisher
Amanda Martin, Executive Publisher
Amy Smith, Associate Editorial Manager
Jeanine Rees, Production Editor
Emely Villavicencio, Senior Graphic Designer
Kylie Bartolome, Licensing Specialist
Natalie Piccotti, Director of Marketing
Kassie Graves, Senior Vice President, Editorial
Alia Bales, Director, Project Editorial and Production

Printed in the United States of America.

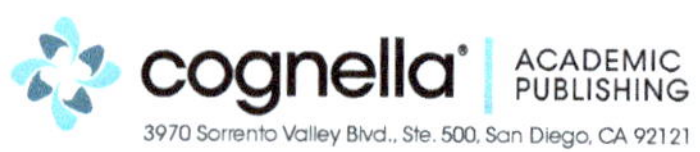

BRIEF CONTENTS

Introduction: Personal Perspective xiii

CHAPTER 1 WHAT IS COACHING? 1

CHAPTER 2 THE COACHING PROCESS 21

CHAPTER 3 TYPES OF COACHING 41

CHAPTER 4 COACHING AS A NURSE LEADER 61

CHAPTER 5 COACHING TO BUILD AND SUSTAIN CAPITAL 77

CHAPTER 6 COACHING TO BUILD LEADERSHIP BEHAVIORS 95

CHAPTER 7 COACHING TO BUILD STRONGER TEAMS 113

CHAPTER 8 COACHING TO BUILD EMPLOYEE DEVELOPMENT (PART I) 127

CHAPTER 9 COACHING TO BUILD EMPLOYEE DEVELOPMENT (PART II) 139

CHAPTER 10 RESOURCES FOR COACHING 153

Index 167

DETAILED CONTENTS

Introduction: Personal Perspective xiii

CHAPTER 1 **WHAT IS COACHING? 1**

Chapter Objectives 1
What Is Coaching? 1
Background and History of Coaching 2
Adult Learning 3
Transformational Learning 3
Behavioral Learning 3
Constructive Development 4
Humanistic 4
Changeology 4
Intended Change 5
Motivational Change 5
Schein's Change 5
Chaos 5
Complex Adaptive Systems 6
Integral Psychology 6
Essential Principles for Coaching 6
Key Aspects for Effective Coaching 8
What Coaching Is *Not* 10
Consulting 10
Mentoring 12
Counseling 14
Teaching 15
Research About Coaching 15
Summary 16
Resources 17
Discussion/Reflection Questions 17
Examples of Coaching Questions 17
References 17

CHAPTER 2 **THE COACHING PROCESS** **21**

Chapter Objectives 21

The Process 21

Problem Identification or Opportunity of Interest (Introductory Session) *21*

Initial Assessment *23*

Coaching *25*

Closure/Celebration *26*

Coaching Plan and Agenda *26*

Coaching Models 29

GROW *29*

OSKAR/OSCAR *30*

CLEAR *31*

Action-Centered Leadership *31*

STEPPPA *32*

SCARF Model *32*

Additional Models *33*

Summary 34

Resources 34

Coaching Agreement/Contract *34*

Worksheet *35*

Discussion/Reflection Questions *38*

Case Example (External and Internal Coaching Perspective) *38*

References 39

CHAPTER 3 **TYPES OF COACHING** **41**

Chapter Objectives 41

Types of Coaching 41

Executive and Leadership Coaching *41*

Career Coaching *43*

Leadership Coaching: Power *44*

Leadership Coaching: Influence *47*

Behavioral Coaching *51*

Strategic Planning Coaching *54*

Team Coaching *55*

High-Performance Culture 57

Summary 57

Resources 58

Discussion/Reflection Questions 58

Worksheet/Table 58

References 59

CHAPTER 4 **COACHING AS A NURSE LEADER 61**

Chapter Objectives 61

Why the Need for a Shift in Leadership Practices? 61

Coaching Mindset 62

Coaching Conversations 64

Feedback Type 65

How to Apply Coaching in the Nurse Leader Role 69

Where and When to Have a Coaching Conversation 70

When Not to Coach 70

Summary 71

Resources 71

Case Example 71

Understanding When to Apply the Coaching Conversation—and When Not To 72

Discussion/Reflection Question: Coaching Culture 73

Real-World Application 74

References 74

CHAPTER 5 **COACHING TO BUILD AND SUSTAIN CAPITAL 77**

Chapter Objectives 77

Types of Capital 77

Human Capital 78

Coaching Culture and Human Capital 79

Requirements for a Coaching Culture 80

Psychological Capital 81

Psychological Capital and Workplace Behaviors 84

PsyCap Development and Coaching 84

Psychological Capital for Nursing and Nursing Leadership Development 87

Summary 89

Resources 89

Discussion/Reflection Question 89

Critical Reflection 89

PsyCap Development Plan: Goal Creation and Pathway Identification 90

References 90

CHAPTER 6 **COACHING TO BUILD LEADERSHIP BEHAVIORS 95**

Chapter Objectives 95

Transformational Leadership 95

Background 96

Building on Transformational Leadership Approach 98

Authentic Leadership 100

Background 100

Situational Leadership 103

Background 103

Coaching Builds Better Leadership Practices 105

Leadership Assessments 107

Summary 108

Resources 108

Discussion/Reflection Questions: Coaching + Leadership 108

References 108

CHAPTER 7 **COACHING TO BUILD STRONGER TEAMS 113**

Chapter Objectives 113

Teamwork 113

High-Performing Teams 114

High-Performing Teams: Professional and Organizational Outcomes 117

Nurse Leaders: Application of Coaching to Build High-Performing Teams 118

GROW 119

ACHIEVE 119

CLEAR 120

OSKAR 120

Interdisciplinary Team Collaboration 121
Nursing Team Development 122
Patient-Centered Care Teams 122
Summary 123
Resources 123
Case Examples 123
References 124

CHAPTER 8 **COACHING TO BUILD EMPLOYEE DEVELOPMENT (PART I) 127**
Chapter Objectives 127
Communication 127
Active Listening 130
Emotional Intelligence 131
Approaches to Improve Communication 134
How to Apply Coaching to Foster Simple, Strong Communication 136
Identify the Problem or Opportunity of Interest 136
Establish Goals 136
Tailor Coaching Plans 136
Consider Group Coaching and Peer Feedback 137
Model and Encourage Reflective Practice 137
Summary 137
Resources 138
Discussion/Reflection Questions 138
References 138

CHAPTER 9 **COACHING TO BUILD EMPLOYEE DEVELOPMENT (PART II) 139**
Chapter Objectives 139
Types of Conflict 139
Interpersonal Conflict 140
Intrapersonal Conflict 140
Task Conflict 140
Types of Conflict Resolution 140
The Five Modes 141
Applying Conflict Management Skills 142

Addressing Conflict Through Coaching 146
Summary 148
Resources 148
Case Example 1: Conflict in a Clinical Setting 148
Case Example 2: Conflict in an Academic Setting 149
Discussion/Reflection Questions 150
References 150

CHAPTER 10 **RESOURCES FOR COACHING 153**
Coaching Programs 153
Books 153
Templates 155
Client/Staff Profile Sheet (Internal Coaching; Leader/Manager as Coach) 156
Internal Coaching Contract Template 156
Coaching Plan Template 158
Action Planning (To Be Completed by Client) 159
Progress Tracker (Based on Action Planning Document) 159
Topic-Based Questions 160
Sites with Online Resources 164
Use of AI and Machine Learning 165
Reference 165

Index 167

INTRODUCTION: PERSONAL PERSPECTIVE

My journey through nursing began like most others, as a staff nurse. My first staff position was in an intensive care unit in a level-one trauma center. During my time there, I wanted to observe and participate in as much as possible. So, I volunteered to serve as a charge nurse, and I collaborated with the unit educator(s) to on-board, teach, and mentor new nurses. I was also part of several shared governance councils—and served as chair for one of them. As time progressed, I developed a deeper desire to teach, develop, and lead incoming nurses, so I decided to seek further education and obtained my master of science in nursing (MSN). Once I received this, I began to teach clinicals then transitioned into academia while obtaining my Doctor of Nursing Practice (DNP) and Doctor of Philosophy (PhD) degrees. Similar to my time in the clinical setting, I engaged in as much activity as possible in academia, which encompassed mentoring, chairing committees, serving in leadership roles (DNP program coordinator, assistant director), and working diligently on my scholarship, focusing on leadership development.

As a Leader

As a leader, I have learned that leadership comes in many forms. I have found that leaders are embedded in every layer of the organization, which has very little—or nothing at all—to do with rank. This may be why some say leadership is a choice, not a rank, and I whole heartedly believe this. While this notion of leadership as a choice undoubtedly helps propel one into a formal or ranked position, I also believe it allows for continual adaptation and adoption of needed leadership behaviors, practices, and skills to move organizations forward; it allows leaders to embrace the evolution of their discipline, lead in the present, and prepare for future.

As a Direct Report

I have spent a lot of time (and still do) as a direct report. During this time, I have been able to observe and absorb leadership behaviors, practices, and skills that positively influenced my personal and professional development. Unfortunately, I also observed many leadership behaviors and practices that negatively influenced my desire to maximize performance and my commitment to the organization. Specific behaviors that I remember were exhibited by those who had little desire to change their approach to leadership—it was very much a traditional or command-and-control approach. Though it worked for some individuals, usually those who were more seasoned or experienced than I was, it was neither effective nor productive for many others. That being said, it wasn't the positive experiences with leadership that inspired me to do my best, but the negative experiences drove me to develop myself to lead in a way that was positive and impactful. During this journey of self-development, I found coaching.

As a Coach

I discovered that when I added an element of coaching to my interactions with students, colleagues, and consulting partners that they were more satisfied with the solutions they self-created than when I directed them toward the solution. While I saw the positive impact coaching had on my clients and colleagues, I didn't realize the added value of applying coaching in day-day interactions. However, once I began to absorb this benefit, it brought heightened awareness to the lack of content presented in nursing leadership textbooks involving coaching. While some graduate-level nursing textbooks do mention coaching, there is little explanation of what coaching actually is and how to apply it, both in general and in critical or challenging situations. Thus, I wrote this book to provide nurses across the discipline with foundational principles of coaching, instructions for applying them in practice, and methods for using these principles to build better leadership practices for themselves and their teams.

CHAPTER 1

WHAT IS COACHING?

Historically, coaching has been viewed as a somewhat punitive or probationary-type process whereby current and emerging leaders receive coaching due to poor performance or lack of insight. However, coaching is anything but punitive or probationary. It is a leadership development tool that can be used to optimize an individual's internal resources, performance, productivity, and overall satisfaction. Like most other professional disciplines, coaching has several renowned organizations promoting their own frameworks, guidelines, and principles of practice. Some organizations include their own code of ethics. These organizations help coaches make coaching a far-reaching tool—one that can extend beyond personal employee growth.

However, before delving into the depth and impact of coaching, as well as the varying models and types, it is important to understand what coaching is, what it isn't, and the theoretical foundations that encompass it.

Chapter Objectives

1. Define coaching
2. Examine the differences between coaching and similar disciplines and professional practices
3. Explore the theoretical underpinnings of coaching

What Is Coaching?

The concept of coaching has many definitions. For example, the International Coaching Federation (ICF), a leading global coaching organization, defines coaching as "partnering with clients in a thought-provoking and creative process that inspires them to maximize their personal and professional potential. The process of coaching often unlocks previously untapped sources of imagination, productivity, and leadership" (ICF, 2023a, para. 5). The Center for Credentialing and Education (CCE) defines coaching as "a career in which professionals have specialized education, training, and experience to assess the needs of clients, collaborate with clients on solutions, and offer strategies that assist individuals and organizations in reaching identified goals" (CCE, 2010, para. 1). The words "offer strategies" in the last sentence of the CCE definition are important to highlight. Offering strategies should be done in a collaborative manner. Next, the International Coaching Community (2023) asserts that coaching is a means to "unlock a person's potential to maximize their performance" (para 2). The last example for inclusion in this text (though there are more) is by Neitlich (2016), chief executive officer (CEO) and founder of the Center for Executive Coaching, and states "coaching is an efficient, high-impact process of dialogue that helps highly performing people improve results that are sustained over time" (p. 13).

These definitions all have the same foundational elements. Thus, coaching in its purest form is an intellectually stimulating dialogue exchange that allows clients to formulate solutions for personal and professional problems. However, this text emphasizes *executive coaching*, which can be viewed as a *leadership development* tool that can be employed to help clients (current or emerging leaders) tap into unrealized potential and identify new opportunities for growth, development, and leadership practices.

Background and History of Coaching

Coaching is a multidisciplinary, multi-theory discipline with contributions stemming from psychology, social science, medicine, leadership, management development, and more (Williams, n.d.). More specifically, the following theories have been identified by the Global Institute of Organizational Coaching (2018) as informing coaching practices:

- Adult learning
- Transformational learning
- Behavioral learning
- Constructive development
- Humanistic
- Changeology
- Intended change
- Motivational change
- Process or Schein's change
- Chaos
- Complex adaptive systems
- Integral psychology

Because coaches may adopt or be guided by a theory based on the type or approach to coaching it is important to have a basic understanding of these theories. Many coaching texts and programs emphasize that coaching borrows mostly from psychology theories, but systems and organizational theories are threaded in as well. Thus, the excerpts below are meant to only provide a snapshot. Additional information about the theories can be explored by reviewing the accompanying web links.

Adult Learning

Just as it sounds, adult learning theory was conceptualized based on the notion that adults learn differently than children. Malcom Knowles pioneered this theory in the 1970s. During his work, he identified six principles of adult learning, including (a) the role of experience, (b) self-directedness, (c) learners' need to know, (d) readiness to learn, (e) orientation to learning, and (f) intrinsic motivation (Conaway & Zorn, 2015). More details of each principle can be further explored at the following site:

https://otpecq.group.uq.edu.au/resources-publications/clinical-educators-resource-kit/approaches-clinical-education/adult-learning-theory

Transformational Learning

The theory of transformational learning was founded by the "father of adult learning" Jack Mezirow, in the late 1970s. His theory aimed to promote development through learning (Wichita State University, 2023). Mezirow outlined 10 phases of learning, including (a) disorienting dilemma, (b) examining self, (c) assessing assumptions, (d) recognizing shared feelings, (e) exploring options, (f) planning a course of action, (g) acquiring knowledge for implementation, (h) provision of trying, (i) building competence and confidence, and (j) reintegrating. More information on the phases can be viewed at the following site:

https://www.wichita.edu/services/mrc/OIR/Pedagogy/Theories/transformative.php

Behavioral Learning

This theoretical perspective embraces the idea that behaviors are learned though interaction with the environment (McLeod, 2023). There are several behaviorists, such as the famous Ivan Pavlov, but John B. Watson, is responsible for igniting the behaviorist movement in the early 1910s. Watson outlined several assumptions or principles of behaviorism, including (a) behavior is learned from the environment, (b) behavior is a result of stimulus-response, (c) psychology should be viewed as a science, (d) behaviorism is concerned with observable behavior, and (e) there is little difference between the learning that occurs in humans and other animals. A more detailed overview can be found at the following link:

https://www.simplypsychology.org/behaviorism.html

Constructive Development

Psychologist Robert Kegan, who built this theory based on the work of Jean Piaget's work in the early 1950s, theorized that adult development focuses on the person's growth and ways of understanding the world (McCauley et al., 2006). Like most theories, constructive development is based on five stages of development, including the (a) impulsive mind, (b) instrumental mind, (c) socialized mind, (d) self-authoring mind, and (e) self-transforming mind. More information on this theory can be found at:

https://learningdiscourses.com/discourse/constructive-developmental-theory/

Humanistic

This theory closely mimics both adult learning theory and constructive theory, suggesting that adults strive for self-actualization. Humanistic theory was founded by Carl Rogers, esteemed psychologist and psychotherapist. He builds on Maslow's hierarchy of needs, connecting learning with the desire of fulfillment of the other needs in the hierarchy (Gandhi & Mukherji, 2023). To learn more, review this resource:

https://www.simplypsychology.org/humanistic.html

Changeology

The Institute of Coaching recognizes John Norcross's transtheoretical model of change, a goal-directed model, which includes five basic steps: (a) psych, (b) prepare, (c) perspire, (d) persevere, and (e) persist. This is a newer theoretical model, but more information can be gleaned from the following resource:

https://www.psychalive.org/video-dr-john-norcross-explains-5-basic-steps-change/

Intended Change

Intended change theory asserts that individuals can engage in purposeful and sustainable transformation with enthusiasm (Boyatzis & McKee, 2006). These sustainable changes occur when individuals focus on the following five major discoveries: (a) the ideal self, (b) the real self, (c); learning agenda, (d) experimenting with and practicing new habits, and (e) developing and maintaining close personal relationships. To learn more, review this resource:

https://onlinelibrary.wiley.com/doi/abs/10.1002/joe.20100

Motivational Change

There are a few different iterations of motivational theory—content and process theories—including Maslow's hierarchy of needs, Alderfer's ERG theory, Herzberg's two-factor theory, and Vroom's expectancy theory (to name a few). However, the basic premise of these theories is that an individual's intrinsic desires or personal needs are different, but the individualized exploration of these desires and needs can unlock motivation. More information on this theory can be found at:

https://upskillcoach.com/blog/theories-of-motivation/

Schein's Change

Schein's (1999) theory considers that change is a psychological dynamic process involving one's one attempt to restructure thoughts, attitudes, and perceptions (Young, 2020). Schein's change theory is based on the widely recognized Lewin's model of change theory. More information can be found here:

https://sites.psu.edu/global/2020/04/07/managing-organizational-change-lewin-schein/

Chaos

Organizational development specialist Margaret Wheatley describes chaos theory as deriving "from the discoveries of 'strange attractors' and fractals. 'Strange attractors' prove that amidst seeming chaos and randomness, patterns evolve revealing an order that is at work in the universe. This evolution is non-linear which means that the slightest variation in the inputs can result in vastly different outputs" (Leadership at Work, 2013, para. 12). In short, organizational behavior may not be that predictable. To read more, view the link below:

https://leadersatworkonline.wordpress.com/2013/05/19/reflections-on-wheatleys-leadership-and-the-new-science/

Complex Adaptive Systems

Complex adaptive systems are a complex, interconnected network of interactions that can adapt and evolve within a respected environment. This theory focuses on the interconnections rather than the individuals. Healthcare systems are considered complex adaptive systems. To learn more, visit this site:

https://bmchealthservres.biomedcentral.com/articles/10.1186/s12913-018-3392-3

Integral Psychology

Pioneered by renowned philosopher Ken Wilber, integral psychology aims to "heal the whole person" by utilizing a comprehensive approach to both human behavior and experiences. This approach draws from the four major forces of psychology: behavioristic, psychoanalytic, humanistic, and transpersonal. More information can be viewed at:

https://www.integralpsychology.org/about-integral-psychology.html

Essential Principles for Coaching

Just as there are many definitions of coaching, there are several schools of thought on "rules" or "foundational principles" of coaching—all of which contain overlapping concepts. For the purposes of this text, which is to provide nurse leaders with a practical guide to coaching, these have been compiled into five essential principles (Center for Creative Leadership, 2023a; Mind Tools Content Team, 2023; Neitlich, 2016; Rogers, 2016). As we look at each of the essential principles, we will refer to the individual being coached as "client."

Essential Principle 1: Create a Safe, Ethical, and Confidential Environment

It is important that the coach create a supportive and nonjudgmental environment for the client (Center for Creative Leadership, 2023a). This helps ensure that the client and the coach are on equal ground and that coaching is not being utilized as a punitive process, but rather a leadership development tool. Affirm that the coaching session is confidential (unless otherwise discussed). Maintain ethical standards by avoiding conflicts of interest and acting in the best interests of the person being coached. This, in turn, will promote trust and respect, both of which are critical to the coach–client relationship, and set the stage for a successful relationship.

Essential Principle 2: Use Coaching to Develop the Client

Coaching is not consulting. Coaches are not in the business of solely offering advice and solutions. Coaching is a client-driven, personalized process that is carefully designed and aimed toward growth and development. Coaches can tap into unrealized potential through skillful, open-ended, Socratic-type questioning, also known as active inquiry. This potential allows the client to develop pathways and solutions for achieving their intended goal. It is important to note that most coaches, especially executive coaches, also offer some sort of additional services, such as training and development activities or exercises to assist their clients in meeting their intended goals. However, coaches should let the client determine what their needs are first. Even if a client wishes to add development, the skillful and open-ended questioning remains steadfast.

Essential Principle 3: Coach the Whole Person

This is a tricky, yet imperative principle. Though coaches may want to solely focus on workplace issues, coaching sessions often bring up personal issues and challenges. Additionally, coaches can expect to see clients having emotional days. While the role of the coach is not to provide therapy, the coach needs to recognize and acknowledge that they're having a conversation with the whole person. Meaning, the coach needs to be aware that emotions and previous experiences will undoubtedly emerge (Mind Tools, 2023). If emotions are too high a coaching session may need to be rescheduled.

Essential Principle 4: Remember the Client is the Resource

Although the coach and client are on equal ground, the client is the one with knowledge of both the internal and external resources available. The client knows how to access these resources; they're resourceful. The coach's role is to build upon the client's resourcefulness.

Essential Principle 5: Work with Coachable Clients

Not all clients are coachable. If a client does not seem open to change, is not committed to improvement, is not open or willing to be on equal footing with the coach, then it will be difficult to establish an effective coaching relationship. Therefore, if a coach determines a client to be unwilling to be coached, it is best to avoid entering a coaching relationship. If a coaching relationship has already been established and progress has not been made related to these issues, it is best to terminate the coaching.

Key Aspects for Effective Coaching

As discussed earlier, coaching is a collaborative and supportive process aimed at helping individuals or teams achieve personal and professional goals. With that said, there are several key aspects that all coaches should include in coaching sessions.

Actively Listening

Coaches must be excellent listeners. They need to fully understand the concerns, needs, and goals of the person being coached. While some sources suggest following an 80-20 rule—the coach should be doing 80% listening and 20% talking—other sources utilize a 70-30 rule. Either way, active listening should be front and center, it enables the coach to be more effective (Ali, 2016; Center for Creative Leadership, 2023b).

Asking Powerful Questions (Active Inquiry)

Asking forward-facing, open-ended questions allows the client to think about the current state versus the desired state without focusing on the past. This type of questioning leads to 'aha' moments. It gives clients the opportunity to dig deep and tap into their own unrealized potential or resources. It helps individuals explore their thoughts, values, and motivations, leading to greater insights and awareness. Powerful questions do not use the word "I." Instead, they should start with "what," "who," "how," and in some situations "why." They should be future-oriented. See the resources section for example questions (Neitlich, 2016; Rogers, 2016; Zentis, 2021).

Establishing Clear Goals and Action Plans

Prior to each coaching session, the client should have a clear and specific goal for each coaching session. With a clear, specific goal in mind, the coach can identify and maintain appropriate direction and purpose for sessions. In some sessions, clients may start out with an intended goal but begin to veer off track. If this happens, the coach can reaffirm the goal of the session and ask the client if they wish to stay with that goal or establish a new goal.

For example, a coach is meeting a client for a 30 minute session. At the start of the session, the coach asks the client what the goal of the session is. The client responds that their goal is to identify two to three ideas for better time management. However, once the session gets started, the client begins to talk about a workplace conflict consuming his workday. The coach would need to say something like, "I am hearing you talk a lot about a conflict in the department. Would you rather discuss this today?" Establishing clear goals for sessions is critical in order for the coach to assist the client in creating an action plan, tracking progress, and measuring success (Neitlich, 2016; Rogers, 2016). Using the earlier example, the client determines that he wishes to discuss the conflict, and the coach reestablishes a goal for the session that includes one key takeaway for better managing the conflict. The client's action plan included utilizing the one key takeaway and practicing it in real time.

The client is ultimately responsible for achieving their desired goals; the coach is there to serve as the intellectually stimulating sounding board, if you will. In general, coaching engagements typically last between 6 and 12 months.

Demonstrating Empathy

Broadly, empathy is demonstrated when an individual is tuned to or sensitive to another's feelings, experiences, or emotions. Because coaching encompasses the whole person, coaches need to be mindful of how the client is feeling. The client may be vocal about a scenario or situation that is currently unfolding, or they may be communicating nonverbally (avoiding eye contact, showing distraction, fidgeting, etc.). Coaches need to recognize and empathize with the client. When coaches display empathy, it shows clients that they matter, which builds better coaching relationships (Positive Coaching Alliance, 2022).

Establishing a Sense of Possibility

Coaches instill a sense of possibility in their clients. They can breed optimism through encouragement, empathetic listening, maintaining forward-facing conversations, and offering support and advocacy during times of uncertainty and change (Neitlich, 2016).

Being Trustworthy

The coach–client relationship is fundamental in determining whether coaching will be successful. The client needs to feel a sense of safety and security when working with the coach. Without trust, it is nearly impossible to have open, honest, and forward-facing conversations. Gauthier (2020), author and master coach, provides the following six, clear techniques that can be helpful in establishing trust in the coach–client relationship:

- Demonstrate a sincere curiosity and interest
- Reassure confidentiality
- Build rapport through body language
- Be 100% mindful
- Be reliable and accountable
- Establish credibility

What Coaching Is *Not*

Now that the definition and elements of coaching have been discussed, it is important to discuss what coaching is *not*. Coaching is not consulting. Coaching is not mentoring. Coaching is not counseling. Coaching is not teaching. Though there are some fundamental similarities between coaching and these related disciplines and professional practices, they are different.

Consulting

Similar to coaching, consulting has many definitions. However, for the purposes of this text, we will only include one, clear-cut, all-encompassing definition, which loosely states that consulting is the business of giving expert advice (Cambridge Dictionary, 2023). Thus, consulting can be viewed as a professional service provided by experts with specialized knowledge and expertise in a particular field. Typically, consultants are hired by businesses, organizations, or governments to provide advice and solutions to specific problems or challenges. Importantly, consulting is conducted utilizing a stepwise approach to achieve key purposes.

Differences Between Coaching and Consulting

In many circumstances, consultants, especially management or organizational consultants have expertise in change management, process, structures, culture, etc. They have industry-specific knowledge (Rogers, 2016). As depicted in the Hierarchy of Consulting Purposes (Turner, 1982), consultants are tasked with identifying and analyzing problems faced by their clients. They serve as the problem-solver, offering customized solutions and/or recommendations. Consultants can also assist with implementation of their recommendations, build organizational support for said recommendations, and provide education to their clients on best practices and current industry trends to facilitate learning, which subsequently influences organizational change. As such, consultants bring their experience, expertise, and outside

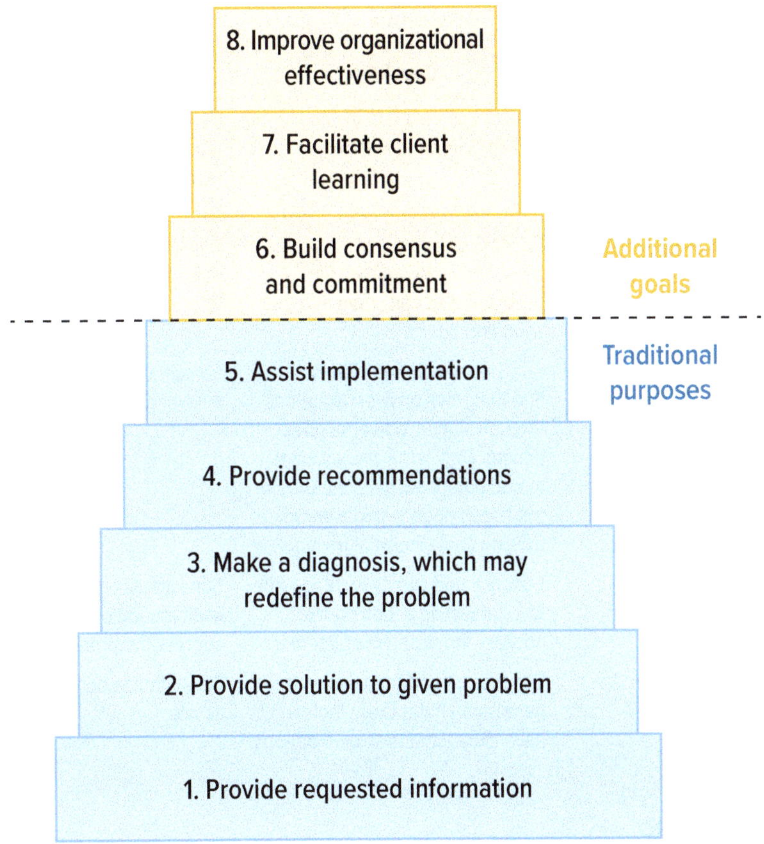

FIGURE 1.1 A Hierarchy of Consulting Purposes

Source: Harvard Business Review, "A Hierarchy of Consulting Purposes," https://hbr.org/1982/09/consulting-is-more-than-giving-advice. Copyright © 1982 by Harvard Business School Publishing.

perspective to help clients solve industry-related problems and achieve their business-related objectives.

Coaches focus on coach–client relationships, working with both personal and professional issues. They work with their client's strengths and weaknesses. They explore factors that are holding clients back from making change (Rogers, 2016), and they create strategies and action plans for goal achievement in a collaborative fashion. Importantly, while coaches do offer advice, they do so with client permission—and after the client has exhausted their options. Table 1.1 further highlights some differences between coaching and consulting (Forbes Coaches Council, 2018).

TABLE 1.1 **Coaching vs. Consulting**

	Coaching	Consulting
Expertise	Coaches are experts in uncovering a client's internal resources.	Consultants are subject matter experts in their respective industry (e.g., IT, finance, etc.).
Diagnosing	Coaches do not diagnose problems. They explore the client's problems and can serve as a sounding board.	Consultants diagnose industry related problems.
Problem-Solving	Coaches encourage clients to find their own answers/solutions through skillful, powerful questioning. *Only* if the client wishes to add additional services should the coach engage in development training (e.g., financial training).	Consultants tell clients the answer to the problem.
Implementation/ Action	Coaches and clients work together to establish an action plan to address the problem of interest.	Consultants create the implementation plan to address the problem.
Advice	Coaches can offer advice with permission if the client feels they have exhausted their own options.	Consultants openly give advice.

Mentoring

Though mentoring and coaching are notably different, the terms "mentoring" and "coaching" can sometimes be used interchangeably. Just like coaching, mentoring has varying definitions. However, an easy-to-digest definition of mentoring offered in this text is provided by the Association for Talent Development (ATD, 2023). ATD (2023) states that mentoring is "a reciprocal and collaborative at-will relationship that most often occurs between a senior and junior employee for the purpose of the mentee's growth, learning, and career development ... Effective mentors often act as role models and sounding boards for their mentee and provide guidance to help them achieve their goals" (para 1).

Mentoring can be informal or formal. For the latter, there are different types of mentoring program options, as well as models. For example, HDRQ, a research-based training company and leading publisher and provider of soft skills training, lists five common mentorship programs, including:

- Career mentoring
- New manager mentoring

- Diversity focused mentoring
- High potential employee mentoring
- Knowledge-sharing mentoring

In brief, career mentoring typically refers to the pairing of a senior executive with a junior employee to offer support and guidance for the mentee's professional development. New manager mentoring allows the newly minted manager to be paired with an individual who can offer advice and guidance to help develop their managerial skills and confidence as a new leader. Diversity-focused mentoring programs allow individuals in underrepresented groups to work with someone to identify and create equitable opportunities for career advancement or development. High potential employee mentoring is a type of mentoring that allows high performers or high potential performers to get the needed support to flourish within the organization. Lastly, knowledge-sharing mentoring refers to the idea of pairing a seasoned employee with a novice employee for a mutually beneficial relationship. The seasoned employee can gain a new perspective on the business or hear new ideas as perceived by the novice employee, while the novice employee can gain insight and wisdom from the seasoned employee. Thus, mentor programs are designed to provide the mentee with advice, knowledge, and support. The ATD includes the following models of mentoring:

- One–one
- Group
- Peer
- Distance or e-mentoring
- Reverse mentoring
- Speed mentoring

With one–one mentoring, the mentor and mentee are the only individuals involved in the mentoring process. Group mentoring occurs when one or more mentors works with a specific group (e.g., youth groups or camps). Peer mentoring occurs when two individuals from the same department are paired to offer support to one another (e.g., department of nursing faculty or cardiac catheterization lab staff nurses). Distance mentoring simply refers to virtual mentoring, which can be done via an online platform like Zoom, Google Meet, TEAMS, or even email. Reverse mentoring occurs when the mentoring model is flipped (e.g., the novice employee is mentoring a seasoned employee) and typically occurs when new applications or technologies are being integrated into the workplace. Speed mentoring usually entails a series of brief conversations and/or questioning with a senior professional. While these different models all bring value to the mentoring process, one–one mentoring is perhaps the most commonly used model.

Counseling

The American Counseling Association (ACA, 2023a) defines counseling as a professional relationship that empowers individuals or groups to achieve their goal for health, wellness, or career. Counselors are licensed professionals who help people overcome issues that lead to turmoil. Such issues can include depression, anxiety, infertility, bereavement, work-related stress, spirituality, trauma, marriage guidance, or relationship issues (National Health Service [NHS], 2020; Rogers, 2016). They collaborate with the client to identify an achievable, manageable, plan of care that mitigates the issue at hand and promotes positive change (ACA, 2023b).

Counseling occurs in multiple stages. These stages, described by Sutton (2021), focus on relationship building, problem assessment, goal setting, counseling intervention, and termination. In the first stage, counselors and clients are learning about one another and scratching the surface on why the client is seeking counseling (Sutton, 2021). Counselors can build rapport with their clients by being mindful of their verbal and nonverbal cues, providing an environment that makes the client feel at ease (e.g., private, calming room), reinforcing confidentiality, and using reflective listening and paraphrasing—to name a few (Lonczak, 2021).

In the second stage, the counselor employs active listening skills while engaging in dialogue with the client to explore their challenges or problems (Sutton, 2021). They aim to draw out specific information regarding the problem, as well as precipitating factors or triggers (e.g., environmental factors, stress levels, time, etc.). In stage three, goal setting, the goals should be created in a collaborative manner and should include clear action steps to help the client meet their goal. Then the counseling intervention can commence. The counselor dictates the type of counseling that will be employed, which is dependent on the client and the situation. Lastly, there is the termination stage. This stage is preplanned in a collaborative manner to promote a positive conclusion with the counseling process.

Learning Checkpoint

Coaching: Shorter term (e.g., 6 to 12 months), more formal in nature, has specific, measurable goals, used for leadership development, and the client finds their solution through powerful, skillful questioning. Coaches can offer advice, if the client desires, after they exhausted their options. Coaches may provide additional services at the request of the client. However, skillful questioning remains the foundation.

Mentoring: Longer term, can be informal or formal, typically conducted with coworkers (e.g., seasoned and novice). Mentors openly *give* advice, typically about the organization, department, or to share the ins and outs of moving up the career ladder.

Counseling: Diagnostic in nature, explores problems that cause emotional distress and require a counseling intervention and an action plan to promote well-being and mental health. Counselors are licensed professionals.

Teaching

Teaching is a multifaceted profession. Teachers are subject matter experts that help students foster their knowledge, skills, and competence in a given subject or subjects. Though traditional teaching typically occurs in schools, colleges, and universities, it can also occur in informal settings such as asynchronous online learning workshops or in hallways during conversations with peers or colleagues. Irrespective of the setting, effective teaching should foster an environment that encourages critical thinking and creativity. This can be achieved through the following seven principles of practice (Carnegie Mellon University, 2023):

1. Acquire relevant knowledge about the students and use that knowledge to inform course design
2. Align the major components of instruction (learning objectives, assessments, and instructional activities)
3. Establish explicit expectations for the learning objective and course policies
4. Prioritize the knowledge and skills that students should focus on.
5. Recognize and overcome expert blind spots
6. Adopt appropriate teaching roles to support learning goals
7. Refine courses or content based on reflection and feedback

Some of the principles may seem similar to those used in coaching. For example, creating learning objectives is similar to creating session goals in coaching. Another example is refining courses or content based on reflection and feedback. In coaching, this would be alternating the action plan to best meet the needs of the client. Although some coaching sessions may require a "teaching" element (e.g., new leader working with a client who desires to build better leadership practices through emotional intelligence development but doesn't understand the foundational principles of emotional intelligence), the sole purpose of coaching is to establish thought-provoking, intellectually stimulating dialogue that results in a collaboratively created action plan that leads clients to their solution.

Research About Coaching

Coaching is a powerful way to develop current and emerging leaders within a variety of settings. Because there is no definitive time frame for applying coaching sessions, coaching is an effective means for leadership and professional development. External or internal coaching can be utilized based on individual and/or organizational needs (externally hired coaches can do 30 to 60 minute client sessions, while internal coaches or managers can coach clients through problems in more frequent, shorter time frames—like micro-coaching sessions.) Coaching can also have financial implications for organizations, with a projected return on investment (ROI) ranging from $4 to $8 for every dollar invested (Neitlich, 2016).

In 2001, Manchester Inc., a global leader in executive coaching programming, surveyed 100 leaders within Fortune 1000 companies who received coaching services. Their study found that the ROI was 5.7 times the investment. Furthermore, coaching was found to have the following benefits from an organizational standpoint: increased productivity, quality, customer service, retention, and cost reduction. From the client perspective, coaching was found to improve working relationships (including relationships with direct reports), teamwork, job satisfaction, conflict reduction, and business relationships with clients (Auerbach, 2023; Shilder, 2019).

Similarly, Marber (2007) of Clear Coaching enlisted 50 organizations to participate in a study exploring the tangible benefits of coaching. Thirty participants completed the study. The following 12 key findings were uncovered and included:

- Increasing perception (63%)
- Acquiring a new skill or improving on an existing one (50%)
- Improving work relationships within a team (50%)
- Being able to see other perspectives (47%)
- Applying some clarity to work life (43%)
- Increasing motivation (43%)
- Having performance approved (43%)
- Resulting in coachee [client] seeming happier (40%)
- Enjoying a better atmosphere (40%)
- Growing into a new role (40%)
- Changing approaches to work situations (37%)
- Reaching agreed-on goals (20%)

Though these studies are dated, these results also align with more current research, from a variety of coaching organizations, coaching practitioners, and talent development groups, with additional benefits showing enhanced self-efficacy, confidence, skill development, behavior change, well-being, and resilience.

Furthermore, coaching is estimated to be a multibillion-dollar industry with projections of steadfast growth into 2030, making it one of the fastest growing disciplines in the world (ICF, 2023b; Willis, 2021). As such, while coaching continues to flourish in both recognition and popularity, coaching organizations, researchers, and practitioners will undoubtedly unveil findings related to the tangible and financial benefits of coaching for both individuals and organizations.

Summary

In this chapter, numerous definitions of coaching were explored, and readers were presented with the definition of *executive coaching*, a *leadership development tool*, that can be employed to help clients (current or emerging leaders) tap into unrealized potential and identify new opportunities for growth, development, and leadership practices. The five essential principles of coaching, as well as the key aspects of effective coaching, set the foundation for Chapter 2.

Resources

Discussion/Reflection Questions

- Explain why it is important to understand the theoretical underpinnings of the coaching profession.
- One key aspect of effective coaching is establishing trust. Provide a detailed example of *how* you can apply Gauthier's (2020), six techniques for establishing trust in the coach–client relationship.

Examples of Coaching Questions

What would you like to discuss during our session today?
What do you want to achieve?
What makes this an important topic?
How will you know you achieved your goal?
What is the benefit of taking action?
What strengths can you utilize to make this change happen?
What are your options moving forward?
What is the first step you can take?
Tell me more.

A list of *some* additional example questions from the University of North Texas (n.d.) can be found here:

https://www.unthsc.edu/culture-and-experience/wp-content/uploads/sites/57/Powerful-Coaching-Questions_-brand.pdf

References

Ali, H. (2016). *What makes a great coach?* International Coaching Federation. https://coachingfederation.org/blog/what-makes-a-great-coach

American Counseling Association (ACA). (2023a). *20/20: Consensus definition of counseling.* https://www.counseling.org/about-us/about-aca/20-20-a-vision-for-the-future-of-counseling/consensus-definition-of-counseling

American Counseling Association (ACA). (2023b). *What is professional counseling?* https://www.counseling.org/aca-community/learn-about-counseling/what-is-counseling#

Association for Talent Development (ATD). (2023). *What is mentoring?* https://www.td.org/talent-development-glossary-terms/what-is-mentoring

Auerbach, J. (2023). *The benefits of business coaching.* College of Executive Coaching. https://www.executivecoachcollege.com/research-and-publications/benefits-of-businesscoaching.php

Boyatzis, R., & McKee, A. (2006). Intentional change. *Journal of Organizational Excellence, 25*(3), 49–60. https://doi.org/10.1002/joe.20100

Cambridge Dictionary. (2023). *Cambridge.org. dictionary.* Retrieved September 6, 2023, from https://dictionary.cambridge.org/us/dictionary/english/consulting

Carnegie Mellon University. (2023). *Teaching principles.* Eberly Center. https://www.cmu.edu/teaching/principles/teaching.html

Center for Creative Leadership. (2023a). *The 6 principles of effective coaching for leaders.* https://www.ccl.org/articles/leading-effectively-articles/the-six-principles-of-leadership-coaching/

Center for Creative Leadership. (2023b). *What is active listening?* https://www.ccl.org/articles/leading-effectively-articles/coaching-others-use-active-listening-skills/#:~:-text=Being%20a%20thoughtful%20listener%2C%20asking,to%20coach%20others%20more%20effectively.

Center for Credentialing and Education (CCE). (2010). *Code of ethics.* https://www.cce-global.org/Assets/Ethics/BCCcodeofethics.pdf

Conaway, W., & Zorn, B. (2015). *The keys to online learning for adults: The six principles of andragogy.* https://www.researchgate.net/publication/299540188_The_Keys_to_Online_Learning_for_Adults_The_Six_Principles_of_Andragogy

Forbes Coaches Council. (2018, June 14). Key differences between coaching and consulting (and how to decide what your business needs). *Forbes.* https://www.forbes.com/sites/forbescoachescouncil/2018/06/14/key-differences-between-coaching-and-consulting-and-how-to-decide-what-your-business-needs/?sh=1b5ba2db3d71

Gauthier, G. (2020, June 8). *6 Techniques to build trust in a coaching relationship.* Go Master Coach. https://www.gomastercoach.com/post/6-techniques-to-build-trust-in-a-coaching-relationship

Gandhi, M. H, & Mukherji, P (2023). Learning theories. In: StatPearls [Internet]. https://www.ncbi.nlm.nih.gov/books/NBK562189/

Global Institute of Organizational Coaching. (2018). *Theories and theorists informing coaching practice.* https://globalioc.com/wp-content/uploads/2018/09/Theories-Underpinning-Coaching-Practice.pdf

International Coaching Community (2023). *What is Coaching?*

International Coaching Federation (ICF). (2023a). *All things coaching.* coachingfederation.org.

International Coaching Federation (ICF). (2023b). *Global coaching study.* https://coachingfederation.org/app/uploads/2023/04/2023ICFGlobalCoachingStudy_ExecutiveSummary.pdf?utm_source=Website&utm_medium=CTR&utm_campaign=GCS&utm_id=Executive+Summary+

Leadership at work. (2013, May 19). *Reflections on Wheatley's leadership and the new science.* https://leadersatworkonline.wordpress.com/2013/05/19/reflections-on-wheatleys-leadership-and-the-new-science/

Lonczak, H. (2021, May 29). How to build rapport with clients: 18 examples & questions. *Positive Psychology*. https://positivepsychology.com/rapport-building/

Marber, J. (2007). *What are the benefits of coaching?* Survey. https://researchportal.coachingfederation.org/Document/Pdf/655.pdf

McCauley, C., Drath, W. H., Palus, C. J., O'Conner, P., & Baker, B. (2006). The use of constructive-developmental theory to advance the understanding of leadership. *The Leadership Quarterly, 17*(6), p. 634–653. doi: https://doi.org/10.1016/j.leaqua.2006.10.006

McLeod, S. (2023, June 27). Behaviorism in psychology. *Simply Psychology*. https://www.simplypsychology.org/behaviorism.html

Mind Tools Content Team. (2023). *What is coaching?* Mind Tools. https://www.mindtools.com/a1plnmq/what-is-coaching

National Health Service (NHS). (2020). *Counselling*. https://www.nhs.uk/mental-health/talking-therapies-medicine-treatments/talking-therapies-and-counselling/counselling/

Neitlich, A. (2016). *The way to coach leaders, executives, and managers*. Center for Executive Coaching.

Positive Coaching Alliance. (2022). *Why coaching with empathy is important*. https://positivecoach.org/the-pca-blog/why-coaching-with-empathy-is-important/#:~:text=An%20empathetic%20coach%20uses%20their,what%20is%20expected%20of%20them

Rogers, J. (2016). *Coaching skills: The definitive guide to being a coach*. McGraw-Hill Education.

Shilder, D. (2019). *Manchester study*. https://www.donnaschilder.com/manchester-study/#:~:text=%E2%80%94%20Manchester's%20coaching%20programs%20delivered%20an,the%20results%20achieved%20through%20coaching

Sutton, J. (2021, July 9). Defining the counseling process and its stages. Positive Psychgology. https://positivepsychology.com/counseling-process/

Turner, A. (1982, September–October). Consulting is more than giving advice. *Harvard Business Review*. https://hbr.org/1982/09/consulting-is-more-than-giving-advice

University of North Texas. (n.d.). *Powerful coaching questions list*. People.

Wichita State University. (2023). *Transformative learning theory*. https://www.wichita.edu/services/mrc/OIR/Pedagogy/Theories/transformative.php

Williams, P. (n.d.). Coaching evolution: From psychological theory to applied behavioral change. *Psychology Alliance, 6*(3), p. 19–22. chrome-extension://efaidnbmnnnibpcajpcglclefindmkaj/https://www.cce-global.org/Assets/BCC/Resources/CoachingEvolution.pdf

Willis, R. (2021, January 4). *3 trends that will shape the future of coaching*. International Coaching Federation. https://coachingfederation.org/blog/3-trends-that-will-shape-the-future-of-coaching

Young, A. (2020, April 7). *Managing organizational change: Lewin & Schein*. Penn State University. https://sites.psu.edu/global/2020/04/07/managing-organizational-change-lewin-schein/

Zentis, N. (2021, January 21). *The importance of coaching questions*. Institute of Organization Development. https://instituteod.com/importance-of-coaching-questions/

CHAPTER 2

THE COACHING PROCESS

This chapter focuses on the coaching process, the workflow of coaching, and the various models of coaching. Though the process and models of coaching overlap, they are distinctly different. Additionally, it is important to note before diving into the chapter content that every coach may have a slightly different process, but the elements included within this chapter are considered the mainstays. Also, the various models that are described are not all inclusive, rather, those included aim to provide coaches with knowledge of the more common, easily applied models during coaching sessions or coaching conversations.

Chapter Objectives

1. Analyze the coaching process
2. Examine the varying models of coaching
3. Articulate the difference between the process of coaching and utilization of a coaching model

The Process

The coaching process is a collaborative and structured process aimed toward developing the client's performance, skills, and leadership, while helping the client achieve their desired goals. Though coaches can develop their own process for coaching, coaching in general should include the exploration of the problem or opportunity (introductory session), an assessment, coaching sessions with check-ins and action planning, and closure/celebration of desired outcomes. Each of these elements is described in more detail in the following sections.

Problem Identification or Opportunity of Interest (Introductory Session)

To effectively coach clients, coaches must have a high-level overview of *why* the client is interested in seeking a coach. This is important for two reasons: (a) to determine if the problem or opportunity of interest is a coachable topic and (b) to get a feel for the coachability of the client. Coaches can explore the problem or opportunity of interest and determine if the client is coachable during an introductory phone call or in-person meeting. The introductory conversation should be casual in tone, but questions should be focused. The following are a few examples of focused questions:

- Tell me why you are seeking a coach.
- Why is this problem or opportunity of interest important to you?
- Are you willing to take action to achieve your goal(s)?
- Are you willing to take accountability for your outcomes?

Though this is a short starter list, the coach will be able to determine whether the client's said problem or opportunity of interest is a coaching issue (e.g., performance improvement, time management, conflict negotiation, etc.) versus a counseling issue (bereavement, home-related stress, etc.). They will also be able to get a feel as to whether or not the client is coachable. For example, there should be red flags if a client's response to bullet point one is something like this: "My boss said I need a coach because I lack vision and strategy. But my boss says that to everyone so, I'm not sold that this is a real issue. But I am seeking coaching to appease him." First, the client doesn't see a problem or opportunity, and second the client is seeking a coach to appease the boss—suggesting they may not be willing to take action or assume accountability for outcomes. In contrast, a coachable client may respond, "I am interested in seeking a coach to help me brand myself to build up my starter company. Right now I feel stuck, but I am willing to try new strategies or software or meet with new people to move the needle forward." In this example, the client is clear in the request for help and displays willingness to take action by trying new strategies. Though not every introductory conversation will be as clear-cut as these two examples, these questions will help the coach to determine if it feels right to move forward with a particular client.

If the coach decides to move forward with the client, it is best to establish a contract. In the contract, it is important to define the scope of the problem or opportunity of interest, incorporate a projected timeline for coaching (duration of sessions), frequency of meeting and delivery method (in person, online, hybrid approach). In addition, the contract will lay out confidentiality and coach–client relationship, as well as ethical obligations (e.g., referring to therapist). Once the contract has been confirmed, the coach can draft the coaching plan based on the client's desires expressed during the introductory session. For managers who wish to utilize a coaching approach, a formal contract is not necessary; however, understanding the process is important for future applications of coaching or if transitioning to an internal coaching position. Importantly, if the client is an emerging or brand-new leader (as is common in healthcare), they may ask for incorporation of development opportunities, and this should be included in the coaching plan. Examples of agreements/contracts can be found in the resource section at the end of the chapter.

Initial Assessment

During the first real meeting with the client, the coach will take a deeper dive into the client's problem or opportunity of interest, identify challenges, objectives, and goals, and review the coaching plan. The coach should conduct (or discuss the plan for) assessment administration, which could include a self-assessment. Other assessments (described below) include CliftonStrengths, Leadership Circle Profile®, Hogan Assessments, DISC® personality assessment, Genos Emotional Intelligence, Myers-Briggs Type Indicator®, verbal 360 assessments, and formal 360 assessments. The coach should also review performance appraisals and job descriptions and schedule a time to observe or shadow the client (Neitlich, 2016). In addition, the coach should introduce or review any online software or paper documents the client may need to access for the coaching duration. Remember, development activities may arise at the request of the client.

CliftonStrengths Assessment

This assessment is quite popular—with over 30 million assessments administered. CliftonStrengths "measures your unique talents—your natural patterns of thinking, feeling and behaving—and categorizes them into the 34 CliftonStrengths themes" (CliftonStrengths, 2023, para. 3). To learn more, visit the following website:

https://www.gallup.com/cliftonstrengths/en/253790/science-of-cliftonstrengths.aspx#ite-254147

https://www.gallup.com/cliftonstrengths/en/253715/34-cliftonstrengths-themes.aspx

Assessment reports include role-specific content associated with the client's CliftonStrengths themes. Some noted benefits of this assessment for leaders include improved awareness of a client's talents, deeper understanding of how a client's strengths shine through in their current leadership role, and heightened awareness of a client's leadership style (CliftonStrengths, 2023).

Leadership Circle Profile

The Leadership Circle Profile® is considered one the most comprehensive 360-degree leadership assessments on the market. According to the Leadership Circle (2025) The Leadership Circle Profile® measures a leaders inner and outer attributes—Creative Competencies and Reactive Tendencies. This allows leaders to gain a new perspective on what they need to develop or leverage to make transformational change. More information on this assessment can be found at this site:

https://leadershipcircle.com/leadership-assessment-tools/leadership-circle-profile/

Hogan Assessments

The Hogan Assessments are personality based, used for both talent acquisition and talent development. For talent development, the assessments are designed to fosterlifelong professional development (Hogan, 2023). Development can focus on leadership, careers, teams, emotional intelligence, or decision-making. To learn more, visit this site:

https://www.hoganassessments.com/talent-development/

DISC

DISC is an acronym for **D**ominance, **I**nfluence, **S**teadiness, and **C**onscientiousness. This personality assessment aims to determine where a client "fits" into the DISC personality profile. Similar to the Hogan Assessments, DISC® has different products that are specific to leadership, team, personal or self-development, workplace, or conflict management (DISC Profile, 2023). To learn more about the DISC® assessments, visit this site:

https://www.discprofile.com/what-is-disc#why

Genos Emotional Intelligence

The Genos Emotional Intelligence assessment is based on the Genos model of emotional intelligence, which includes six competencies: (a) self-awareness, (b) awareness of others, (c) authenticity, (d) emotional reasoning, (e) self-management, and (f) positive influence *or* inspiring performance (depending on assessment selected). This assessment is unique because it includes both internal and external benchmarks in the report, provides an evidence-based interventions workbook for building emotional intelligence, and provides two separate models for those on the front lines (nurses) and those in formal leadership roles. To learn more about the Genos emotional intelligence model or assessment, visit "Emotionally Intelligent Leadership" at Genos International (2023) at the following link:

https://www.genosinternational.com/leadership/

Myers-Briggs Type Indicator

Myers-Briggs personality assessments are perhaps the most well-known on the market. This assessment includes four personality preference pairs, including extraversion or introversion, sensing or intuition, thinking or feeling, and judging or perceiving. The Myers-Briggs aims to enhance a leader's development from a personal and organizational perspective—including supporting teams and conflict management (The Myers-Briggs Company, 2023). More information on the Myers-Briggs assessments can be viewed at Myers-Briggs Type Indicator® (MBTI®):

https://www.themyersbriggs.com/en-US/Products-and-Services/Myers-Briggs

Additional Assessments

The aforementioned assessments are just an example of the numerous assessments that are available to coaches. Coaches need to explore the varying assessment tools and seek certification for administration and debriefing, or work with a third party to administer and debrief results (e.g., Summit Assessment Solutions).

Coaching

Once the client has completed their assessment, the coach should arrange a session to debrief their results. During the debrief, the client will have the opportunity to review their results, seek clarification on interpretation of results, and validate self-assessment findings with those from peers, colleagues, and superiors. From this point, the coach and client can establish a more formal coaching plan to assist the client with meeting their goal by reestablishing the big picture. Remember, the coaching occurs while posing those skillful, powerful, open-ended questions or active inquiry. During this part of the coaching process, coaches can integrate their own preferred model of coaching to guide the sessions.

Results Check-in and Action Planning

Equally important to posing those skillful, powerful questions is tracking results. In order to track results, coaches can employ a variety of methods, including utilization of the objectives and key results approach, SMART goals, impact mapping, 360-assessments, business outcome measurements, and rating personal metrics or self-assessments (Forbes Coaches Council, 2022a). Tracking results and adjusting the coaching plan as necessary is a critical component for client success.

Holding clients accountable is also essential for success. Coaches can help hold clients accountable by revisiting the client's progress on the action steps that were planned in the previous session. Although the client may have developed clear, actionable steps, it is not uncommon for clients to stall or not commit to their action plan. According to the Center for Executive Coaching (2023), clients may lack commitment due to (a) not being serious about the goal, (b) not accurately calibrating how much work it will take to achieve the goal, (c) not wanting to do the work required to be successful, (d) not having the skills or knowledge to take the action he said he would take, (e) having time management issues, (f) shifting the focus of coaching due to a bigger priority emerging, or (g) having limiting beliefs or fears that stand in the way of success. When lack of commitment occurs, the coach must explore the reasons why by utilizing active inquiry. The barriers or challenges uncovered during the active inquiry process may require the client to shift goals until those challenges or barriers are resolved.

Closure/Celebration

When the client has achieved their goal(s), celebrate the win! The celebration should not be formal in nature (e.g., lunch/dinner, cocktails and hors d'oeuvres), but the coach should ask the client to share their emotions on the success, ask the client how they would like to celebrate, and of course, the coach should also share their own enthusiasm and positivity. Though the celebration marks a closure of the planned goal(s), it is a good point for the coach to explore the client's next steps. Likely, the organization has moved to explore new initiatives, or new problems or opportunities have emerged for the client, leaving room for additional coaching services.

Coaching Plan and Agenda

Though coaches may have their own template for coaching plans, below is a simple coaching plan template that can be adapted to suit individual client needs. Table 2.1 presents an example for a client who wants to build on their leadership abilities.

TABLE 2.1 **Coaching Plan**

Session		Actions	Development Activities
1. Initial meeting	Further explore problem or opportunity of interest. Confirm coachability of the client. Establish agreement. Review the coaching plan and make changes as needed. Set goals. Plan for assessment administration. Introduce *or* review any online software the client may need to access (e.g., online assessments, coach's website for development activities, etc.)	Take assessments. Explore online software as necessary.	None this week.
2. Review assessments	Give client time to review assessments. Debrief results, discuss how findings fit into the big picture and specific goals. Confirm coaching plan.	Establish plans of action and metrics.	Activities suggested at client's request. Could include topics such psychological capital, emotional intelligence, effective leadership, change leadership, team mobilization, etc. Topics can be client-specific and created as needed.
3–7. Coaching	Coaching begins and continues weekly or biweekly (depending on sessions in contract).	Implement action plans created during coaching sessions.	Same as above.
8+. Coaching	Coaching continues. Result check-ins are built into the remaining sessions to ensure clients are on target to meet their goals or to determine whether the goals changed.	Adjust coaching plan as necessary to ensure client is on track to meet their goal(s).	Same as above.

(Continued)

TABLE 2.1 **Coaching Plan (*Continued*)**

Session		Actions	Development Activities
XX. Closure	As outlined in the contract, this is the last session (though it could be renewed/modified based on client needs). Discuss where the client is in terms of their goal (they may be a few weeks shy of meeting it or they may have achieved it).	Celebrate achieved goals and explore future opportunities for working with the client. Continue working with client on current goal(s) if needed.	Same as above.
Continue building/modifying this plan according to client needs.			

Note. This is a modifiable, easy-to-use sample coaching plan.

In addition to coaching plans, coaches should also create session agendas such as that given in Table 2.2. Coaches can schedule 60 to 90 minutes for client sessions weekly or biweekly to start. Session frequency can be reduced based on progress (e.g., monthly). It is worth noting that coaching sessions are guided by coaching models, which will be introduced in the following section.

TABLE 2.2 **Coaching Session Agenda**

Time	Topic
XX	Recap any events that have occurred since the last meeting. • Clarify/address any areas of concern or interest.
XX	Inquire about plans of action (e.g., if client established points of action from last session, see if those were completed). • Inquire about takeaway points (e.g., what did they find valuable).
XX	Topic inquiry for the scheduled session (this should be established at the start of each session) • If the client has more than one item to discuss, prioritize the items; there may not be enough time in the session to cover both. If there is, great. If not, the topic of most importance was explored.
XX	Outcomes (what does the client hope to achieve in this session). • What metrics would they like to establish for measuring success?
XX	Coaching on topic—this is the bulk of the session.
XX	Closing (establish how the client wants to move forward with the information gleaned from the session. They should have a clear plan of action to carry forward.

Note. This is a modifiable example coaching agenda. The XX denotes suggested time to spend on each topic. This is at the discretion of the coach and depends on the total time frame of the session, but typically only lasts for a few minutes (e.g., 5 to 10 minutes). The bulk of the time should be dedicated to coaching.

In summary, the coaching process refers to the structured process that the coach and client follow during the coaching engagement. It is individualized and adaptable to meet the needs of the client. As denoted above, the process begins with the exploration of the problem or opportunity of interest and progresses through to closure in a stepwise approach.

Learning Checkpoint

- The coaching process is collaborative and structured, aimed toward client development; it is the workflow
- In the coaching portion of the process, coaches can integrate their desired model to facilitate the sessions

Coaching Models

Coaching models are comprised of theoretical or conceptual frameworks that coaches use to guide their practice. There are a variety of models, but some of the most commonly utilized models for executive coaching include GROW, OSKAR/OSCAR, CLEAR, Action-Centered Leadership, STEPPPA, and SCARF (Forbes Coaches Council, 2022b). You will notice that the initial steps in some of the models mirror the first steps in the coaching process (e.g., contracting, establishing/reestablishing the big picture). Each of these common models are described in more detail below

GROW

The GROW model was introduced in the 1980s by Graham Alexander, Alan Fine, and Sir John Whitmore, all of whom were business coaches. It is perhaps one of the most well-known coaching models. The GROW acronym stands for:

- **G**oal
- **R**eality
- **O**ptions (or obstacles)
- **W**ill (what will you do or way forward)

To apply this model in coaching practice, the coach would first establish a goal (ensuring that it is specific and measurable). Next, the coach would examine the client's current reality. To do this, the coach would ask one or more pointed questions. For example, "Where are you now in terms of this goal." Then the coach would explore all possible options for achieving this goal. Again, the coach can ask pointed questions, or they may engage in a brainstorming session to help the client come up with as many options as possible. Lastly, the coach needs to work with the client to achieve a pathway for achieving their goal (Mind Tools Content Team, 2023c; Rogers, 2016). To learn more, visit the following website:

https://www.mindtools.com/an0fzpz/the-grow-model-of-coaching-and-mentoring

OSKAR/OSCAR

OSKAR was developed by Paul Jackson and Mark McKergow in the early 2000s as a solutions-based approach to coaching. This model has been hailed as one of the best models of coaching (Forbes Coaches Council, 2022b). The acronym OSKAR stands for:

- **O**utcome
- **S**cale
- **K**now-how
- **A**ffirm/Action
- **R**eview

The outcome is what the client hopes to achieve from the session. The client measures how close they are to achieving the goal on a scale, usually from 1 to 10. The know-how is understanding the client's current state versus desired state, where the coach and client discuss how to bridge the gap. In the affirm/action step, the coach affirms the positive qualities or aspects they have observed, and they continue to build on what works. Lastly, review is exactly as it sounds—the coach and client review the outcomes from the actions and determine whether further action is needed. Interestingly, there is a variation of the OSKAR model, which is the OSCAR model, by Karen Whittleworth and Andrew Gilbert. In the OSCAR, the acronym stands for:

- **O**utcome
- **S**ituation
- **C**hoices/Consequences
- **A**ctions
- **R**eview

This model is quite similar, with the notable difference being the choices/consequences. In this step, the coach "helps the client generate as many alternative courses of actions as possible, increasing their awareness about the consequences (upsides and downsides) of each choice, including the practicality, cost, fit with client's values and so on" (Rogers, 2016, p. 100). To read more about this model visit the following website:

https://www.mindtools.com/agrk092/the-oskar-coaching-framework

https://www.revolutionlearning.co.uk/article/the-oscar-coaching-model/

CLEAR

Developed by Peter Hawkins, the CLEAR model aims to create transformational change over a multi-session engagement (Forbes Coaches Council, 2022b). The acronym in this model stands for:

- **C**ontract
- **L**isten
- **E**xplore
- **A**ction
- **R**eview

During the contracting step, coaches should discuss the ground rules for the coaching agreement and determine the outcomes desired by the client or organization. Next, the coach should be actively listening during the coaching sessions to help the client gain perspective into their current situation. Exploring involves deeper exploration of the situation to help clients understand the impact of the situation and challenge current assumptions surrounding the situation. Next, the coach and client can work collaboratively to develop a clear, specific set of action steps for addressing the situation. Lastly, during the review step, coaches should review the client's progress and continue to assist the client in identifying pathways to achieve their desired goals.

Action-Centered Leadership

Action-centered leadership (also known as the three circles model) was pioneered by leadership theorist John Adair in the early 1970s. This model emphasizes three main areas for leaders to focus on: (a) task achievement, (b) team information and management, and (c) individual development (Mind Tools Content Team, 2023a). Task achievement enables the coach to take a deeper look at the client's leadership role and abilities. This step helps the client identify their goals. In the second step, the coach helps the client focus on developing strong team dynamics (e.g., communicating, navigating conflict, having crucial conversations, etc.). In the third step, clients are challenged to identify/address each of their team member's unique needs.

Understanding each member's needs, desires, or areas of growth contributes to a more successful team. More about this model can be viewed at Action Centered Leadership™ "The Three Circles Model: Balancing Task, Team and Individual Focus":

https://www.mindtools.com/aghzl5f/action-centered-leadership

STEPPPA

In the early 2000s, Angus McLeod conceptualized the STEPPPA model. This model stands for:

- **S**ubject
- **T**arget
- **E**motion
- **P**erception
- **P**lan
- **P**ace
- **A**ction

The subject is exactly that—exploring what subject or topic the client wishes to be coached on. The target step requires clients to identify a clear, measurable, attainable goal (incorporating a SMART goal framework is helpful when working with clients to create goals). Emotion is a unique aspect to this model, with a "life coach" feel. Nevertheless, in this model, it is believed that emotions drive behaviors and actions. Therefore, understanding a client's feelings or emotions surrounding a situation or problem can be quite helpful in assisting them with planning their actions. Perception allows the client to sit back and digest their big picture, which is a nice segue to the plan step. During the planning step, clients and coaches collaboratively draft reasonable, attainable plans of action for achieving the desired goal. Act refers to the client acting on their plan, making adjustments as necessary if emotions or perception change.

SCARF Model

Developed in 2008 by David Rock, the SCARF model aim to influence behavior in social situations (Mind Tools Content Team, 2023b). The acronym stands for:

- **S**tatus
- **C**ertainty
- **A**utonomy
- **R**elatedness
- **F**airness

Status, in this model, simply refers to the client's need to feel important to others. Certainty refers to the client's confidence or ability to determine current or future situations. Autonomy looks at the client's ability to make their own decisions. Relatedness describes how the client feels working with others (e.g., is there some type of bond or relationship). Lastly, fairness is how the client perceives others' treatment or response to their needs or suggestions. More information on this model can be found in the book *Coaching Skills* by Jenny Rogers (2016) or the following website article "David Rock's SCARF Model: Using Neuroscience to Work Effectively With Others" by Mind Tools Content Team (2023b):

https://www.mindtools.com/akswgc0/david-rocks-scarf-model

Additional Models

There are a variety of coaching models, some outside the aim of this text, but two additional coaching models are worth mentioning: HILDA and LAEDAN. The HILDA model follows a simplistic, conversational approach and can be easily applied to any coaching scenario (remember, coaching is an intellectually stimulating *dialogue exchange* that allows clients to formulate solutions for personal and professional problems). The HILDA acronym refers to:

Highlight—Coaches address the client's issue at hand.

Identify strengths—Coaches should inquire about their client's strengths, attributes, and skills.

Look at possibilities—Coaches should explore the client's pathways for achieving their goal.

Decide and commit—Clients should decide how they wish to achieve their goal (derived from the pathway conversation in the previous step).

Analyze—Identify metrics for knowing when the client has achieved success (e.g., improved 360-degree leadership assessment).

As coaches test frameworks to guide their practice, they may find that certain elements of different frameworks work best for their client population. For example, the author of this text and executive coach and leadership trainer for current and emerging nurse leaders uses a self-created conceptual model that works best in this population, the LAEDAN model. In this model, the acronym stands for:

Learning—Exploring the client's problem or opportunities of interest; establishing a big picture with the client.

Assessing—Determining where the client is currently versus their desired state. This is achieved through both informal and formal assessment measures and confirms the coaching plan.

Engaging—Engaging in active inquiry (asking the client forward-facing, powerful questions).

Developing—Forming clear, specific action plans with the client.

Adjusting—Checking in with client to track their progress; adjusting plans as necessary.

Noting—Reflecting on and celebrating achievement(s)and collaborating on next initiative (if applicable).

Other models can be found at this website:

https://uk.sagepub.com/sites/default/files/upm-binaries/26777_01_Allison_&_Harbour_CH_01.pdf

Summary

The coaching process is the workflow outlining the necessary steps or stages that will guide the coaching engagement. The coaching model refers to the theoretical or conceptual framework that coaches use during the coaching process to facilitate effective coaching. Importantly, coaches can select a model based on their coaching experience, style, preference, and client needs—or they can conceptualize a model of their own.

Resources

Coaching Agreement/Contract

Review the following resources:

SampleCoachingAgreement.pdf

https://uk.sagepub.com/sites/default/files/template_for_coaching_contract.pdf

Based on your review (and from the viewpoint of an *external* coach), create a coaching agreement, using a template/format of your choice for the following client:
New nurse manager of a 45-bed emergency department within a level I trauma center.

- Client has never been in a formal leadership role and desires to engage in a combination of coaching and development to bolster her leadership skills.

Worksheet

Review the coaching plan below (this was also included on Table 2.1). Using the blank template, create a *detailed* coaching plan, including how to further explore the problem or opportunity of interest, type of assessment(s), framework for establishing goals (e.g., SMART goal framework), development topic and activities, how the development activities will occur (online, during sessions, combination of both), metrics for measuring success, and closing session for the same client—the new nurse manager of a 45-bed emergency department within a level I trauma center. Client has never been in a formal leadership role and desires to engage in a combination of coaching and development to bolster her leadership skills.

Session		Actions	Development Activities
1. Initial meeting	Further explore problem or opportunity of interest. Confirm coachability of the client. Review the coaching plan and make changes as needed. Set goals. Plan for assessment administration. Introduce *or* review any online software that the client may need to access (e.g., online assessments, coach's website for development activities, etc.)	Take assessments. Explore online software as necessary.	None this week.

(Continued)

Session		Actions	Development Activities
2. Review assessments	Give client time to review assessments. Debrief results, discuss how findings fit into the big picture and specific goals. Confirm coaching plan.	Establish plans of action and metrics.	Activities suggested at client's request. Could include topics such psychological capital, emotional intelligence, effective leadership, change leadership, team mobilization, etc. Topics can be client-specific and created as needed.
3–7. Coaching	Coaching begins and continues weekly or biweekly (depending on sessions in contract).	Implement action plans created during coaching sessions.	Same as above.
8+. Coaching	Coaching continues. Result check-ins are built into the remaining sessions to ensure clients are on target to meet their goals or to determine whether the goals changed.	Adjust coaching plan as necessary to ensure client is on track to meet their goal(s).	Same as above.
XX. Closure	As outlined in the contract, this is the last session (though it could be renewed/modified based on client needs). Discuss where the client is in terms of their goal (they may be a few weeks shy of meeting it *or* they may have achieved it).	Celebrate achieved goals and explore future opportunities for working with the client. Continue working with client on current goal(s) if needed.	Same as above.
Continue building/modifying this plan according to client needs.			

Session		Actions	Development Activities

Discussion/Reflection Questions

Now that you have created a coaching agreement and coaching plan for the new nurse manger with assessments and debriefing completed, you can begin the most important part of the process—coaching. Based on your review of the coaching models presented in this chapter, select one model that you would like to use with your client. Explain how this model relates and differs from the other models presented and explain why you chose this model and why you think it would work for the nurse manager client.

Using the same nurse manager client, create a list of 10 open-ended, thought-provoking questions that could be useful (in any session) during the coaching engagement. This is a good opportunity to practice forward-facing, intellectually stimulating questions that may be useful for future clients.

Case Example (External and Internal Coaching Perspective)

Penelope is a certified nurse practitioner working in an outpatient setting. She has been a nurse practitioner for 5 years. Prior to this, she worked in the intensive care unit for nearly 9 years and assumed a leadership role during that time frame. Though Penelope has had a successful 5-year tenure as a nurse practitioner, she feels a strong desire to return to a less clinical, more leadership focused role within her current outpatient setting—a role that will be available in future months. However, she fears her lack of collegial connection and "dusty" leadership knowledge and skills will be looked at in a negative light and could interfere with her gaining the role.

What else does the coach need to learn from Penelope before an agreement can be put in place?

If Penelope asks for development opportunities with her coaching, what type of development would be best for her?

What assessment measure would be of value in this engagement?*

What metrics would be valuable to measure when working with Penelope?

*Assessment and metrics can look slightly different for *internal* coaches or those coaching from a management position because they may not be certified to administer the assessments and/or they may not have a relationship with a subcontractor to administer the assessments. However, it is still important to be familiar with the varying assessments.

References

Center for Executive Coaching. (2023). *How to coach clients to be accountable.* How to coach clients to be accountable - Center for Executive Coaching

CliftonStrengths. (2023). *Live your best life using your strengths.* https://www.gallup.com/cliftonstrengths/en/252137/home.aspx

DISC Profile. (2023). *What is DISC?* https://www.discprofile.com/what-is-disc#why

Forbes Coaches Council. (2022a, January 4). How 12 coaches quantify results and prove their worth to clients. *Forbes.* https://www.forbes.com/sites/forbescoachescouncil/2022/01/04/how-12-coaches-quantify-results-and-prove-their-worth-to-clients/?sh=34760f007006

Forbes Coaches Council. (2022b, October 27). 5 executive coaching models used by the best coaches. *Forbes.* https://councils.forbes.com/blog/best-executive-coaching-models

GENOS International. (2023). Emotionally intelligent leadership. https://www.genosinternational.com/leadership/

Hogan. (2023). *Do people really know their workplace reputation?* https://www.hoganassessments.com/talent-development/

Leadership Circle. (2025). *Leadership circle profile.* https://leadershipcircle.com/leadership-assessment-tools/leadership-circle-profile/

Mind Tools Content Team. (2023a). *Action-centered leadership.* Mind Tools. Action Centered Leadership™ - The Three Circles Model: Balancing Task, Team and Individual Focus (mindtools.com)

Mind Tools Content Team. (2023b). *David Rock's SCARF model: Using neuroscience to work effectively with others.* Mind Tools. https://www.mindtools.com/akswgc0/david-rocks-scarf-model

Mind Tools Content Team. (2023c). *The GROW model of coaching and mentoring.* Mind Tools. https://www.mindtools.com/an0fzpz/the-grow-model-of-coaching-and-mentoring

The Myers-Briggs Company. (2023). *Myers-Briggs Type Indicator®*. Official Myers Briggs Personality Test. themyersbriggs.com

Neitlich, A. (2016). *The way to coach leaders, executives, and managers*. Center for Executive Coaching.

Rogers, J. (2016). *Coaching skills: The definitive guide to being a coach*. McGraw-Hill Education.

CHAPTER 3

TYPES OF COACHING

This chapter will discuss the varying types of coaching that fall under the umbrella of executive coaching, including career, power and influence, behavioral, team, and high-performance culture coaching. While this is not an exhaustive list, these commonly seen types are particularly relevant to healthcare leadership growth and development.

Chapter Objectives

1. Examine the varying types of coaching
2. Examine executive coaching vs. leadership coaching terminology
3. Explore active inquiry approaches to the types of coaching discussed

Types of Coaching

Our world endorses many different types of coaching, including those in the popular categories of life, wellness, spiritual, relationship, and executive coaching. Since the purpose of this text is to provide nurse leaders with a practical guide for executive coaching, this chapter will focus on varying subtypes of executive coaching, also considered a coach's niche.

Executive and Leadership Coaching

Historically, executive coaching was aimed toward developing the most senior and executive leaders, including senior vice presidents (SVP), vice presidents (VP), and of course, CEOs. However, it has since evolved to encompass middle managers and emerging leaders (Rogers, 2016). As a result, varying types of coaching emerged—all still under the umbrella of executive coaching.

It is important to note that some coaches differentiate executive coaching and leadership coaching based on their client's position (e.g., "executive coaching" when working with those in high-level positions and "leadership coaching" when working with current middle managers and emerging leaders) or the topic of inquiry because some topics do tend to be more executive in nature (e.g., strategic planning). Other coaches use the terms "executive coaching" and "leadership coaching" interchangeably because executive coaching does, after all, stem from a need for *leadership growth and development.*

As an executive coach for current and emerging nurse leaders, I was hesitant to use the term "executive coaching," fearing the term "executive" would sound as if it only applied to the highest-level leaders. I have since come to learn that once people understand the end goal (leadership development), the term doesn't really matter. Nevertheless, for those who wish to differentiate the verbiage based on the topic or client population (e.g., chief nurse executive (CNE), chief nursing officer (CNO), or director of nursing), Table 3.1 provides a visual of how/when a coach could use "executive coaching" versus "leadership coaching" terminology. This is not an exhaustive list.

As depicted in the table, there is substantial overlap between the two types of coaching, which is why some coaches use the terms interchangeably.

TABLE 3.1 Executive Coaching vs. Leadership Coaching Terminology

	Executive Coaching	Leadership Coaching
Audience	VP, SVP, CEO, COO, CIO, CNE, CNO	Middle management, emerging leaders
Topic of Inquiry	**Common Coaching Topics for Executive Leaders:** 1. Emotional intelligence 2. Power and influence 3. Managing transitions 4. Articulation and fluency (e.g., communication skills) 5. Executive presence 6. Negotiation 7. Building high-performing teams 8. Tactical, deliberate, and systematic thinking 9. Succession planning	**Common Coaching Topics for Middle/Upper Management:** 1. Emotional intelligence 2. Leadership presence 3. Articulation and fluency (e.g., communication skills) 4. Conflict resolution/ negotiation 5. Building strong teams 6. Change management 7. Succession planning 8. Time management
Assessments	CliftonStrengths Genos Emotional Intelligence Hogan Assessments Leadership Circle Profile® Myers-Briggs Type Indicator® DISC personality assessment® (This is not an all-inclusive list.)	CliftonStrengths Genos Emotional Intelligence Hogan Assessments Leadership Circle Profile® Myers-Briggs Type Indicator® DISC personality assessment® (This is not an all-inclusive list.)
Organizational Impact	Development aligns with organization's strategic goals	Development aligns with organization's strategic goals
Goals	Could be specific to the executive's current role, responsibilities, or direct challenges	Could be specific to the leader's current role, responsibilities, or direct challenges; could also be more general in nature and applied to different situations (e.g., time management)

Irrespective of the terminology used, executive coaching is a highly individualized and effective development process aimed toward improving the skills and attributes and leadership competencies of current and emerging leaders. As such, many business and healthcare organizations incorporate or offer executive coaching as part of leadership development for their current and emerging leaders. Even more recently, large nursing organizations such as the American Organization for Nursing Leadership (AONL) have called for a "shift in mindset" to establish a more coaching-based leadership approach for nursing leaders (more on this can be found in Chapter 4).

Career Coaching

Career coaching helps clients prepare for and/or explore professional growth opportunities. Coaches who specialize in career coaching could help clients refresh their curriculum vitae or resume, enhance their interviewing skills/behaviors, or aid with the transitioning process when entering a new position or organization (Eisler, 2021; Lyons, 2022). In addition to including the key aspects of coaching, which were discussed in Chapter 1 and include: (a) active listening, (b) asking powerful questions (active inquiry), (c) establishing clear goals and action plans, (d) having empathy, (e) conveying a sense of possibility, and (f) being trustworthy, career coaching has a few additional aspects to consider. These include but are not limited to job search strategy skills, interviewing role play, or helping clients identify an entire new career path. If coaching internal employees, the coach should have insight into organization trajectories/pathways for promotion.

Career coaching still employs asking powerful, open-ended questions (active inquiry), that focuses on the client's big picture or dream (Neitlich, 2016). Some questions career coaches may ask could include the following:

- What is your dream job?
- What are the obstacles in obtaining your dream job?
- What do you love about what you do now?
- What don't you love about what you are doing now?
- What is important to you?
- What are you passionate about?
- What are your strengths?
- What do you want in terms of your career?
- What don't you want in terms of your career?
- What are your accomplishments?
- What type of career (or work) excites you?
- What type of career (or work) is off-putting?

Leadership Coaching: Power

Power and influence are interesting elements of leadership. Power can be viewed as having the capacity or ability to yield actions from others based on one's positional authority (George Washington University, 2024). Power can have a negative connotation, which is why some leaders (current or emerging) don't strive for or exert their power. Forbes Coaches Council member Melissa Eisler (2021) beautifully summarizes this concept:

> In order to use power for good, you first have to have power. This may sound obvious, but it is often what do-gooders get wrong and where they fail. They reject power, labeling it as a manipulative and dirty concept. Yet, without power, they are far more limited in the good they can bring to their organizations and to the world (para. 1).

Power, when used correctly, can have far-reaching and impactful results, creating positive and sustainable change. One cannot create change without power (Gibson, 2022). For a current or emerging leader to use power in an effective and positive way, it is important to have an understanding of the dynamics of power and know that a combination approach is what drives change. French and Raven (1959) explored the complexities of power and identified the following five bases of power: (a) reward, (b) legitimate, (c) referent, (d) expert, and (e) coercive (French and Raven, 1959, as cited by Kovach, 2020; Mind Tools Content Team, 2023a).

Reward

The reward power base refers to a leader's ability to extend rewards to direct reports (e.g., promotions, salary raises, development opportunities, etc.). When leaders exert this type of power, there is a high likelihood that direct reports will execute the tasks/responsibilities that are asked of them. However, there are notable limitations to solely focusing on this type of power. Nursing managers, for example, have the ability to operate off a reward base—to a degree. They can create desirable assignments for staff and provide meaningful recognition and praise, pacifying staff for a period of time. However, there will be a time when direct reports no longer value the rewards, and power is weakened in return (Mind Tools Content Team, 2023a). Additionally, it is rare for middle or even senior managers to exert sole control over salary increases or promotions, so these types of rewards, which may hold more weight, cannot be utilized.

Legitimate

Legitimate power, also known as authority, refers to the power one holds in their current organization and according to the organization's hierarchy

(Center for Leadership Studies, 2023; Kovach, 2020). Examples of individuals with legitimate power include CEOs, chief medical officers (CMOs), and CNEs. These individuals have the ability to hire, terminate, and influence promotions, salary increases, and creation of new positions. Though legitimate power can be used to gain additional power (e.g., gaining more direct reports or new teams), one's scope of power is narrowed (Mind Tools Content Team, 2023a; Kovach, 2020). For instance, the CMOs impact on nursing is less than it is on medicine. Additionally, legitimate power can be unstable, particularly in a financially fragile system where organizational restructuring may result in eliminated or merged positions. Once the position of authority is eliminated, so is the power, which was a by-product of the position.

Referent

Referent power is based on earned respect and/or admiration (Kovach, 2020). Those with referent power are leaders who are attractive or likable in some way, whether that is because of their personality, vision, energy, or leadership style (Kovach, 2020). They tend to be influential. Celebrities provide an example of a referent power. They can influence everyday consumers to purchase certain drinks buy specific brands of clothes and even vote a certain way with their endorsement (Mind Tools Content Team, 2023a). In the workplace, direct reports, or even colleagues, may be swayed by this type of power, so it is critical for leaders to maintain a keen self-awareness of their values, integrity, and ethical decision-making to ensure personal gain does not overtake collegiality or workplace relationships. Leaders should use this type of power as a managerial tool to create strong teams, satisfaction, and productivity.

Importantly, referent power is not limited to current leaders—it can illuminate through emerging leaders as well. As noted by Kovach (2020), those in informal leadership roles who yield the likability or admiration factor that is the foundation of referent power, can be influential in creating pleasant work environments, building a culture of trust and knowledge sharing, setting them up for success when they do enter a more formal or executive leadership role. This is especially true for nurses, who are often promoted to leadership positions based on clinical practice expertise and professional/collegial relationships.

Expert

Those with expert power are considered subject matter experts. Their knowledge and expertise grants their credibility and power (Mind Tools Content Team, 2023a; Pennsylvania State University, 2023). Similar to referent power, one does not need to be in a formal leadership role to exert expert power. Expert power is found across the disciplines, and it is critical to organizational success, especially in healthcare, where expert knowledge is imperative for the day-to-day operations of the health system.

The notion that nurses yield expert power may be surprising to some, given the varied, and sometimes broad field of nursing. Thus, it is worth a brief revisit to Benner's novice to expert nursing theory. According to this theory, which boasts five steps—novice, advanced beginner, competent, proficient, and expert—nurses achieve "expertise" when they can recognize and capitalize on resources around them to attain their goals (Nursing Theory, 2023). A nurse's knowledge and experience influence their ability to have a broad vision, function in fluid situations, and maintain the delivery of safe, quality, care (Ozdemir, 2019). Their continued education and practice experience feed their expertise. Moreover, for nurses working in specialized units or departments, expertise can be further demonstrated through advanced training and certifications (e.g., stroke certified registered nurse, certified nurse manager and leader, nurse executive advanced-board certified nurse executive-board certified, etc.). Thus, nurses should capitalize on both their referent and expert power when advocating or engaging in change endeavors.

Coercive

Broadly, coercion is the act or practice of forcing participation or persuading one to do something to produce a favorable outcome by employing threats, force, or other means. Coercive power is no different; someone in a position of power is securing favorable participation or results based on threats, force, or other coercive measures. Kovach (2020, p. 6) identified several ways coercive power can be used, which include the following:

- Public or workplace shaming
- Refraining from sharing relevant/important information
- Excluding one from meetings (or other workplace events)
- Purposefully damaging or inflicting poor results on a project
- Not approving time off
- Harassing
- Threatening termination
- Withholding workplace rewards (bonuses, paid time off)

Though coercion power is overwhelmingly negative in terms of the impact on employees and potential legal issues, there are *some* circumstances where coercive-*type* power can be used. For example, a nurse confides in her nurse leader that she aspires to assume the assistant manager position. Yet, she is habitually late and sometimes speaks inappropriately with her orientees. This employee could benefit from coercive-*type* power. This can be employed by holding a one-to-one with the nurse, sharing observations and any other direct evidence regarding the late clock-ins and orientee feedback. Reinform her of the responsibilities and expectations of the assistant manager role, and highlight that without change, it will be difficult to support her application for this leadership role.

Informational Power

Informational power was not part of the original five bases, but it was added several years later. Informational power refers to one's ability to have control over information that other people deem valuable. Some examples include having inside knowledge of organizational or department finances or impending layoffs or organizational restructuring (Mind Tools Content Team, 2023a). Informational power quickly dissipates once the "need to know" information has been disseminated to interested parties (Best, 2020).

Personal Power

Understanding the varying types of power, potential consequences, and outcomes of such are necessary element of nursing leadership. Even more so, for nursing leaders who wish to help their staff, patients, or colleagues meet their own goals, they should build their own power base. Huston (2008) highlighted 11 strategies for building a personal power base, which include the following:

- Becoming an expert
- Identifying positive role models and seek mentoring relationships
- Networking and building coalitions
- Maintaining the freedom of maneuverability
- Being self-aware (leadership styles play a role here)
- Staying focused on goals
- Choosing your battles carefully
- Being willing to take risks
- Giving up some ego
- Working hard and being a team player
- Taking care of yourself

Though Huston's work is dated, many of these strategies are reflected in present practice—especially the building of networks and coalitions. Identifying and strategizing how to better capitalize on or foster current networks is a well-recognized development exercise for both current and emerging leaders. A quick resource/tip sheet for how to do this can be accessed here:

https://coachingfederation.org/blog/power-bases-leadership-tool

Leadership Coaching: Influence

Influence, another essential component of leadership, can be defined as having the capacity to "affect [and] change how someone or something develops, behaves, or thinks" (Cambridge Dictionary, 2023). Research on influencing behaviors has been well documented in the literature, spanning over 30 years and leading to the identification of 11 influence tactics. These tactics are categorized by soft and hard (Feser, n.d.; Lee et al., 2017; Sisti, 2014) and will be further described below.

Influence Tactics: Hard and Soft

The tactics discussed in this text are based on a meta-analytic review of influence tactics by Lee et al. (2017) and can be separated into soft or hard tactics. Soft tactics are those that can be employed without causing harm to relationships (Mind Tools Content Team, 2023b). Conversely, hard tactics are those that may *potentially* negatively impact relationships—it depends on the application. Soft tactics include rational persuasion, appraising, inspirational appeals, consultation, exchange, and collaboration. Hard tactics include legitimation, coalition, pressure, ingratiation, and personal appeals.

The Soft Tactic of Rational Persuasion

Rational persuasion involves the presentation of data, clear facts, and logical argument among a target group (colleagues, staff, or peers) to elicit a favorable response to a proposal or request (Lee et al., 2017; Mind Tools Content Team, 2023b). Typically, leaders capitalize on their expertise, experience, and use of visual elements (charts, graphs, etc.) to support their argument. Rational persuasion can be an extremely effective technique when used with a target group that perceives the leader as trustworthy and shares a similar mindset. Feser (n.d.) provides common statements by a leader using rational persuasion, including "Given the data available, the most logical approach is ..." or "the company's transformation is necessary to achieve growth, to reduce costs, and to beat the competition ..." (p. 7)

The Soft Tactic of Exchange

Exchange involves favor-swapping. It is based on reciprocity. This means a leader can influence a target individual through the exchange of favors. This tactic falls in the line with the idea "If you do this, I will do that." Using the exchange tactic in a work-related situation may look something like, "If you run my 4 p.m. meeting today, I will run your 9 a.m. tomorrow," or "if you support my proposal at tomorrow's meeting, I will support yours in next month's meeting." Basic principles of favor-swapping; producing a win–win for both parties.

The Soft Tactic of Consultation

Consultation requires leaders to ask individuals or target groups for input and active participation to help with goal achievement for a proposal, project, or change process. This tactic, though simple and straightforward, has shown to bolster an individual's sense of control and ownership over the proposal, project, or change process, leading to commitment (Lee et al., 2017). Feser (n.d., p. 7) provides examples of common statements by leaders who use consultation tactics, including "in your opinion, what would be the advantages and disadvantages," and "My suggestion is XYZ. What would you suggest?"

The Soft Tactic of Inspirational Appeals

Inspirational appeals refer to a leader's ability to gain buy-in by appealing to an individual or target group's values, hopes, ideals, or emotions. These appeals produce enthusiasm and enhance confidence among individuals (Lee et al., 2017; Mind Tools Content Team, 2023b). Inspirational appeals can be an influential tactic; however, it does require a leader to know an individual or target group's values and motivators.

The Soft Tactic of Appraising

As noted by Lee et al. (2017, para. 22), "appraising is the practice of explaining how fulfilling a request or supporting a proposal will produce personal benefit or help to progress the target's career." Though appraising still utilizes logical argument and presentation of data, this tactic uses extrinsic motivation to elicit an individual or target community's involvement with a proposal or project (Mind Tools Content Team, 2023b).

The Soft Tactic of Collaboration

With collaboration, the emphasis is placed on offering the necessary resources and assistance to individuals or target groups to complete a requested task. Though this may seem similar to exchange, collaboration offers the *means* for an individual or target group to accomplish the desired goal, whereas exchange is more focused on favor-swapping (Lee et al., 2017). Essentially, collaboration tactics make it easier for persons to complete the task at hand.

The Hard Tactic of Legitimating

Legitimation functions from a complex requesting style, with the leader adding rationalization for their command-and-control approach to leading (Feser, n.d.). This approach is used when a leader aims to exert their authority. Feser (n.d.) states that leaders who reference laws, rules, or directives in their requests are exercising legitimating tactics. Some common statements from leaders using this tactic may begin like these: "According to policy, all air travel must ..." or "As you know, it is a standard practice that ..." (Feser, n.d., p. 4). This tactic is similar to legitimate power in the sense that individuals or target group decisions are influenced simply because of their leader's authority or role (Mind Tools Content Team, 2023b).

The Hard Tactic of Coalition

Coalition refers to a leader's ability to enlist others to help them influence an individual or target community. They need the help of others to achieve a goal they could not complete on their own (Feser, n.d.). Coalition complements the notion that there is power in numbers. An example of a coalition could be a group of middle management intensive care unit nurse leaders working together to influence a senior leader's position on implementing a nurse leader institute.

The Hard Tactic of Pressure

Pressure tactics entail the use of threats, repeated reminders, or aggressive actions to influence an individual or target group (Lee et al., 2017). Pressure tactics go hand in hand with bullying. And literature demonstrates that bullying can yield a plethora of negative outcomes, both on the individual being bullied and the organization at large.

The Hard Tactic of Ingratiation

In simple terms, ingratiation uses the concept of "buttering up" before making a request. Though flattery and praise can be well received by individuals and target groups, if it is used with ill will or manipulative intentions, this tactic can harm relationships and raise suspicions of the leader's authenticity. However, if used correctly and with good intent, this can be a successful tactic.

The Hard Tactic of Personal Appeals

Personal appeals are based on the notion that an individual or target group is asked to carry out a project, request, or proposal out of loyalty, trust, or friendship (Freser, n.d.). Freser (n.d.) notes typical statements used by leaders employing a personal appeal, which can include "Can I count on you guys for making ..." or "You and I go back a long time in this company, I'd really like your help on ..." Similar to ingratiation, if this tactic is overused or used with deceptive intentions, it can make an individual or target group feel manipulated, and result in resentment (Mind Tools Content Team, 2023b).

Power and influence coaching focus on building current and emerging leaders' ability to lead with impact. Some key aspects of power and influence, as well as coaching exploration tips, can be viewed in Table 3.2.

TABLE 3.2 Aspects of Power and Influence Coaching

Power and Influence Topics	Coaching Exploration Entails ...
Sources of power	Helping clients harness their sources of power (e.g., expertise, relationships, network, role, etc.).
Influence tactics	Exploring the client's go-to influence tactics; identifying new strategies; uncovering opportunities for execution of said strategies.
Self-awareness	Developing the client's self-awareness; where they are now in terms of what power and influence they hold.
Relationships	Exploring/identifying, quality rating, and leveraging relationships that can move the client and organization forward.
Conflict resolution	Exploring current conflicts, identifying strategies to reduce conflict, incorporating role-play if necessary.
Leading change	Narrowing in on power base, influence strategies, relationships internal and external to organization, and mapping out engagement ideas to mobilize employees.
Emotional intelligence	Exploring awareness of self and others to optimize influence.
Communication	Optimizing communication to appeal to the audience (e.g., not all individuals or groups should be presented to in the same way. Explore message delivery—emotion, facts, data, and justification should be altered to match target groups for maximum effectiveness).
Negotiation	Exploring/improving negotiation skills to optimize success of influence and improve power base.

Thus, the goal of power and influence coaching is to capitalize on leadership effectiveness, achieve organizational goals, and inspire innovation. Like other forms of coaching, power and influence coaching enlists the use of self and 360-degree assessments, role-play of real-world scenarios, and identification of outside development opportunities that can help the client build, refine, or maximize their power base and influence tactics.

Behavioral Coaching

Behavioral coaching is one of the most interesting types of coaching because it can be threaded into just about every aspect of coaching. For example, clients engaged in leadership coaching may identify one or more behaviors that need to be improved or eliminated. The same applies to power and influence coaching—there is usually a behavior that needs improvement (e.g., verbal and nonverbal communication, overtalking, interrupting, or overpowering staff, or poor response to constructive feedback). Marshall Goldsmith, a nationally recognized guru in behavioral coaching, believes that behavioral coaching is not only valuable to top executives, but it's an equally valuable tool for future leaders (Goldsmith, n.d.).

Because behaviors are often habitual, behavioral coaching focuses on establishing new habits to improve or eliminate behaviors, all based on behavior frameworks, chains, or theories. However, creating new habits is often challenging—it takes time, practice, and a desire to change. Road bumps or transient failures are inevitable, but persevering with a positive mindset will lead to success.

Andrew Neitlich teaches about behavior coaching by setting the stage with a relatable and popular behavior chain—that is, Noom (the weight loss program), which is a great way to visualize how behavior change works. Consider this weight loss program. It incorporates psychology-driven practices (behavior change) to help users change their eating habits (Figure 3.1).

In this behavior chain, users identify their triggers (e.g., dinner party with favorite foods), work through their immediate thoughts (e.g., to eat or not to

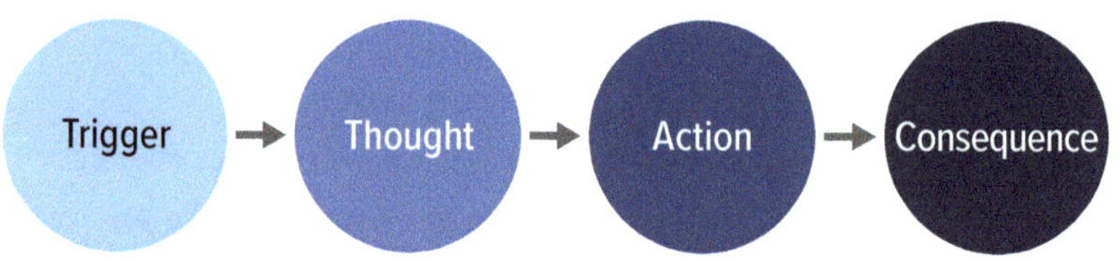

FIGURE 3.1 Noom Behavior Chain

Source: Noom, "Noom Behavior Chain," https://www.noom.com/blog/behavior-change-101-the-behavior-chain/. Copyright © 2023 by Noom, Inc.

eat), engage in an action (e.g., actually eat or not eat), and understand the consequence to the action (e.g., when eating two plates of desserts induces nausea, the desire to repeat this behavior is decreased). Coaches highlight the notion that every day will not be a success, but rather an opportunity to identify areas of change to apply in future days. This approach has been so successful that Noom is now expanding their behavior change platform to appeal to those with chronic health conditions, such as hypertension and diabetes (Noom, 2023).

Another example that can be applied to behavior change is Ivan Pavlov's two-step approach. Pavlov, the Nobel Prize winning physiologist, is well recognized for his experiment with classical conditioning or stimulus and response. Though Pavlov's research was done with dogs, many psychologists believe that conditioning is a form of learning that can be used to influence people (Neitlich, 2016; Rehman et al., 2023). For instance, when leaders model positive, effective principles or behaviors among colleagues, teams, or staff, positive results will ensue (Kouzes & Posner, 2017). Think of this as stimulus (modeling effective leadership behaviors) and response (increased job satisfaction, productivity, organizational culture, etc.).

Nurse leaders can utilize a similar approach to help change the behaviors of their current lower-level management—assistant directors, supervisors, and emerging leaders. Because nurse leaders do not typically have the privilege of coaching their clients for 45 to 60 minutes each week or biweekly, adapting a streamlined and effective approach is critical. One way of doing this would be to identify the current behavior and informally, while on-the-job, help the client work toward creating a new behavior or response.

Identify Behavior

Identifying a behavior that needs to be improved or eliminated is the first step. The coach should advise the client that wishes to make a behavior change to choose only one behavior. The selected behavior should be both specific and measurable, such as encouraging their direct reports more, eliminating interrupting, providing constructive criticism in private, or using a calm tone of voice, etc. (Neitlich, 2016). Selecting one specific and measurable behavior will help both the coach and the client track and monitor progress and feedback from colleagues and direct reports about the chosen behavior.

Create New Behavior or Response

As with the Noom program example above, and most other behavioral-based programs, behavior change takes time to root. Thus, coaches and clients should not expect a new behavior to become an established behavior for several months. When helping a client make a new behavior or response part of the everyday routine, a stepwise approach can be of great value. Neitlich (2016) highlights his stepwise approach to helping clients turn new behaviors into habits, which includes taking detailed notes about what occurred when the client implemented their new behavior. Probing questions in this phase should be simple and straightforward (e.g., What worked? What didn't?). Asking these probing questions can help the coach and client redirect. In Neitlich's (2016) second phase, he builds in monthly 360-degree assessments to measure how often the client exhibited the new behavior. The client will determine as one of their goals the target number for positive consecutive 360-assessments reporting the new behavior. For nurses, either formal 360-assessments or informal 360-assessments can be utilized. Lastly, because behavior change ebbs and flows, it is critical to maintain the coaching relationship to help the client stay on track.

In summary, behavioral coaching focuses on helping individuals identify and improve or eliminate a behavior that could be limiting personal or professional growth. As previously discussed, behavioral change does not happen overnight; in fact, most behavior changes require several months to a year of consistent practice.

Learning Checkpoint

Match the type of coaching to the appropriate description.

Career	a. No impact on relationships
Power Reward Legitimate Referent Expert Coercive Informational	b. Having the right (or desired) information c. Securing participation based on threats or force d. Subject matter experts e. Can be threaded into any aspect of coaching f. Based on admiration g. Yielding authority h. Allows for the exploration of professional growth opportunities
Influence Positive tactics Hard tactics	i. Negatively influences relationships j. Ability to extend reward(s)
Behavior	

Strategic Planning Coaching

Though this text is geared toward equipping nurse leaders with tools and tips to coach their clients (employees in most cases) and to foster growth and development (rather than coaching executive leaders on strategic planning), it is important to have some *basic* understanding of strategic planning in the event a client is serving as a staff contributor for the strategic planning committee. Strategic planning is typically an executive-level leadership activity used to identify short-term and long-term organizational priorities, allocate resources, strengthen operations, and determine organizational direction (Cote, 2020).

Strategic planning occurs in a stepwise approach. One of the earliest steps in strategic planning is strategy formation. In this step, organizations will begin with an in-depth evaluation of the current situation by performing internal and external assessments (CFI, 2025; Waxman & Knighten, 2023). Typically, these assessments include an environmental evaluation and a strengths, weaknesses, opportunities, and threats (SWOT) analysis. Once these assessments have been completed, the leadership team will discuss the findings and formulate strategies that move the organization forward and align with the mission, vision, and values of the organization (Waxman & Knighten, 2023).

More information on these assessments can be viewed here:

https://www.shrm.org/resourcesandtools/tools-and-samples/hr-qa/pages/basics-of-environmental-scanning.aspx

https://corporatefinanceinstitute.com/resources/management/swot-analysis/

The next step is strategy implementation. Strategy implementation can be more complex because it requires both tactical planning and budgeting considerations prior to the actual implementation. This may include allocation of resources, upcoming fiscal year financial planning, etc. (CFI, 2025; Waxman & Knighten, 2023). Most importantly, executive leadership should have clear communication with all stakeholders to gain buy-in prior to actual implementation in order to optimize success.

Lastly, ongoing strategy evaluation is necessary to ensure that the initiative is performing at its intended expectation (CFI, 2025). CFI (2025) lists three activities necessary for strategy evaluation, including "reviewing the internal and external factors affecting the implementation of the strategy, measuring performance, and taking corrective steps to make the strategy more effective" (para. 9). Leadership can use a variety of methods to monitor performance, including personal dashboards and snapshot reviews (Waxman & Knighten, 2023).

More information on strategic planning can be accessed here:

https://balancedscorecard.org/strategic-planning-basics/

Team Coaching

Team coaching functions on the same principles as standard coaching, with team coaching involving more than one client at a time. Team coaching focuses on improving the effectiveness, performance, and cohesion of a team. It is designed to help teams work together more efficiently, communicate better, and achieve their collective goals. Team coaching also hones in on the *team's* functionality by exploring the attributes, intrapersonal awareness, relationships, and collective experiences (Leading Effectively Staff, 2023). As stated by Siang and Canning (2023, para. 1) "teams are the engine of the corporate machine. They bring together diverse sets of skills to solve problems, innovate, and execute strategy." Thus, a strong team is a necessity for organizational success. As such, team coaching has become in high demand for most organizations (ICF, 2025), resulting in the creation of a specific set of coaching competencies and specialty certification. The team coaching competencies can be viewed here:

https://coachingfederation.org/credentials-and-standards/team-coaching/competencies

The nurse leader–coach should first identify the type of team. There are several types of teams in healthcare organizations, a few of which include core teams (direct patient care providers), coordinating teams (resource managers for the core team), contingency teams (groups designed to manage specific events), ancillary service teams, and support services and administration teams (Sanford et al. 2024). Nurse leaders, however, typically work with core teams within their respective department. Nevertheless, once the team has been identified, assessments should be administered, coaching engagements should follow, and a post-coaching assessment should be used to measure growth. An additional team coaching resource article can be viewed here:

https://researchportal.coachingfederation.org/Document/Pdf/3000.pdf

Some key aspects to consider with team coaching can be viewed in Table 3.3.

TABLE 3.3 Team Coaching Considerations

The need for team coaching	Coaches should have a firm understanding of why team coaching is warranted (e.g., optimize patient safety or satisfaction scores, implement new procedure change that requires a team-based approach, improve site visits, etc.).
Team assessment administration and results review	Conduct a team assessment (interviews, observation). Administer assessments (e.g., Team Diagnostic survey, Five Dysfunctions of a Team, OR self-create based on publicly available tools*). Review all data from assessments. *An excellent resource is the New York Times best-selling team leadership text by Patrick Lencioni entitled: The Five Dysfunctions of a Team: A Leadership Fable
Team coaching	Explore team goals and team dynamics. Highlight the need for accountability, build in exercises to capitalize on team strengths, work through weaknesses, and formulate agreements on how the team will work together to tackle upcoming projects, initiatives, communication improvement or conflict resolution. Build in development opportunities and role-play to simulate site visits, team procedure changes, or critical conversations for peer-to-peer development. Team coaching may also involve coaching team leaders on how to lead their teams more effectively. Some elements of this may include: • enhancing emotional intelligence • clearly articulating expectations for behavior, performance, or future development • understanding the complexity of the triad: individuals, team, and organization at large More information available at https://www.ccl.org/articles/leading-effectively-articles/the-dynamics-of-team-coaching/
Team reassessment and evaluation	Evaluate growth and development by administering a post-coaching assessment.

High-Performance Culture

Leadership influences culture. Therefore, before leaders begin to emphasize and coach clients on high-performing cultures, they must realize that they are the ones who set the stage. Some critical leadership elements for setting the stage include emotional intelligence, clear and effective communication, ability to recognize and capitalize on human capital as well as display a team attitude and utilize a coaching style of leadership. As imagined, some leaders may have exceptional insight as to where they stand with the aforementioned leadership elements, while others have a blind spot—or blind spots. Nonetheless, if leaders want high-performing cultures, they need to start by evaluating their own leadership abilities and identify areas of improvement. To do this, leaders can complete their own self-assessment, conduct informal 360 assessments or request more formal 360 assessments. Then, they can work with their human resource counterparts for development opportunities within the institution, or they can work with their own coach. Once areas of improvement have been identified or narrowed, leaders can begin to put their plans for improvement into action. During this time, leaders should continue to gather assessment data from peers and direct reports, as well as their own self-assessments, so that progress can be monitored. Modeling growth, development, and commitment to personal excellence is the impetus for cultivating a high-performing culture; it will inspire a collective mentality (Performance Consultants, 2025).

After the self-assessment and development has been modeled, leaders can move into assessing their organizational culture. As with any assessment, this can be done with surveys, observations, or interviews. The purpose is for the leader as the coach to establish the current state versus the desired state and effectively communicate desired organizational behaviors, values, expectations, and key performance indicators. High-performance culture coaching should also explore employee engagement and motivation—investigate the inspiration. It should also encompass effective performance management strategies (e.g., establishing clear, measurable goals, receiving feedback, reinforcing accountability, etc.) and metric evaluation. Building a high-performance culture does entail a long-term, close and collaborative effort with the client and organization at large because expectations may change and financial stability may wax or wane, hindering or promoting change within departments. Nevertheless, high-performance coaching, when successful and consistent, can improve productivity, satisfaction, and innovation.

Summary

The types of coaching encompassed within executive coaching are vast. As leaders, a foundational knowledge of these types, as well as their applicability to fostering the growth and development of clients, is paramount to modeling a coaching style of leadership, especially in nursing. The next chapter will detail the nurse as coach.

Resources

Discussion/Reflection Questions

You are approached by one of your direct reports, Michael, who holds a supervisory role on the night shift. He is concerned about the lack of respect he is receiving from some of the regular night shift staff. Upon further inquiry, Michael states that he feels powerless and wants to identify where he can grow and develop his power base. How can you, as the leader–coach, help Michael develop his power base?

Your assistant manager approaches you to discuss how she can improve her leadership behaviors. Succinctly describe how you, as the leader–coach, can help her establish new behaviors and track results.

Worksheet/Table

Based on the prompt below, please write what area within executive coaching would be most applicable to the growth and development of the client (more than one area can be applicable):

A client looking to improve their active listening: ________________
A client wanting to build better relationships with their team: ________________
A leader who wants to build a stronger culture: ________________
A client who wants to yield more influence: ________________
A client who wishes to improve their leadership presence: ________________
A leader who wants to build better leadership practices: ________________
A client who needs to bolster their communication skills: ________________
A leader who needs help with negotiation: ________________

References

Best, K. (2020). *Power bases: A great tool for the leadership coach.* International Coaching Federation. https://coachingfederation.org/blog/power-bases-leadership-tool

Cambridge Dictionary. (2023). *Cambridge.org dictionary.* https://dictionary.cambridge.org/us/dictionary/english/influence

The Center for Leadership Studies. (2023). *What is legitimate power?* https://situational.com/blog/what-is-legitimate-power/

Corporate Finance Institute. (2025). Strategic planning. https://corporatefinanceinstitute.com/resources/management/strategic-planning/

Cote, C. (2020, October). *Why strategic planning is important.* Harvard Business School Online. https://online.hbs.edu/blog/post/why-is-strategic-planning-important

Eisler, M. (2021, August 25). Four ways leaders can use power for good in the workplace. Forbes Coaches Council. *Forbes.* https://www.forbes.com/sites/forbescoachescouncil/2021/08/25/four-ways-leaders-can-use-power-for-good-in-the-workplace/

Feser, C. (n.d.). *When execution isn't enough.* https://www.mckinsey.com/~/media/mckinsey/featured%20insights/leadership/when%20execution%20isnt%20enough/when-execution-isnt-enough-chapter-3.pdf

George Washington University (2024). *Team dynamics: Dealing with power and influence.* Himmelfarb Health Science Library. https://guides.himmelfarb.gwu.edu/teamdynamics

Gibson, K. (2022, May). *4 ways to gain power and influence to lead change.* Harvard Business School Online. https://online.hbs.edu/blog/post/how-to-gain-power

Goldsmith, M. (n.d.). *Coaching for behavioral change.* Marshall Goldsmith.

Huston, C. (2008). Eleven strategies for building a personal power base. *Nursing Management.* https://downloads.lww.com/wolterskluwer_vitalstream_com/journal_library/nmg_07446314_2008_39_4_58.pdf

International Coaching Federation. (2025). ICF Announces new team coaching offerings. https://coachingfederation.org/blog/icf-announces-new-team-coaching-offerings

Kouzes, J., & Posner, B. (2017). *The leadership challenge: How to make extraordinary things happen in organizations* (6th ed). Wiley.

Kovach, M. (2020). Leader influence: A research review of French & Raven's (1959) power dynamics. *The Journal of Values-Based Leadership, 13*(2), https://scholar.valpo.edu/cgi/viewcontent.cgi?article=1312&context=jvbl

Leading Effectively Staff. (2023). *The dynamics of team coaching.* Center for Creative Leadership. https://www.ccl.org/articles/leading-effectively-articles/the-dynamics-of-team-coaching/

Lee, S., Han, S., Cheong, M., Kim, S., & Yun, S. (2017). How do I get my way? A meta-analytic review of research on influence tactics. *The leadership Quarterly, 28* (1), 210–228. doi: https://doi.org/10.1016/j.leaqua.2016.11.001

Lyons, M. (2022, February). Do you need a career coach? *Harvard Business Review.* https://hbr.org/2022/02/do-you-need-a-career-coach

Mind Tools Content Team. (2023a). *French and Raven's five forms of power.* Mind Tools. https://www.mindtools.com/abwzix3/french-and-ravens-five-forms-of-power

Mind Tools Content Team. (2023b). *Yukl and Tracey's influences*. Mind Tools. https://www.mindtools.com/a3nll0k/yukl-and-traceys-influencers

Neitlich, A. (2016). *The way to coach leaders, executives, and managers*. Center for Executive Coaching.

Noom. (2023). *About us*. https://www.noom.com/about-us/

Nursing Theory. (2023). *From novice to expert*. https://nursing-theory.org/theories-and-models/from-novice-to-expert.php

Ozdemir, N. (2019). The development of nurses' individualized care perceptions and practices: Benner's novice to expert model perspective. *International Journal of Caring Sciences, 12*(2), 1279–1285. https://internationaljournalofcaringsciences.org/docs/81_ozdemir_special_12_2.pdf

Pennsylvania State University. (2023). *Taxonomy of social power*. Penn State World Campus. https://courses.worldcampus.psu.edu/welcome/psych485/001/content/07_lesson/05_pag.html

Performance Consultants. (2025). *High-performance cultures*. https://www.performance-consultants.com/what-we-do/high-performance-cultures/

Rehman, I., Mahabadi, N., Sanvictores. T., & Rehman, C. (2023). *Classical conditioning*. StatPearls. https://www.ncbi.nlm.nih.gov/books/NBK470326/

Rogers, J. (2016). *Coaching skills: The definitive guide to being a coach*. McGraw-Hill Education.

Sanford, N., Lavelle, M., Markiewicz, O., Reedy, G., Rafferty, D. A. M., Darzi, L. A., & Anderson, J. E. (2024). Decoding healthcare teamwork: a typology of hospital teams. *Journal of Interprofessional Care, 38*(4), 602–611. https://doi.org/10.1080/13561820.2024.2343835

Siang, S., & Canning, M. (2023, February 23). *Coaching your teams as a collective makes it stronger*. Harvard Business Review. https://hbr.org/2023/02/coaching-your-team-as-a-collective-makes-it-stronger

Sisti, K. (March, 2014). *Influence tactics*. Penn State. https://sites.psu.edu/leadership/2014/03/02/influence-tactics-2/

Waxman, K., & Knighten, M.L. (2023). *Financial and business management for the doctor of nursing practice* (*3rd ed.*). Springer Publisher.

CHAPTER 4

COACHING AS A NURSE LEADER

This chapter will emphasize the many responsibilities of the nurse leader. Readers will be prompted to reflect on their own leadership experiences—both as a leader and as a direct report. This chapter will begin to form the connection between the nurse leader's role and coaching.

Chapter Objectives

1. Explore the need for a new shift in leadership
2. Examine feedback models/frameworks
3. Analyze when/how to apply a coaching conversation

Why the Need for a Shift in Leadership Practices?

Present-day leaders are working in complex environments, whether that is within a healthcare system or higher education—though some might say it's more like complex chaos with fluctuating financial realities, changing cultures, and continuing evolution of technology (Albert et al., 2022). Rapid advancement of technology has been shown to benefit health systems and nurse leaders at large through improved managerial processes (e.g., data tracking, monitoring, report logging), and it also has positively impacted patient care through reduced medication errors, improved tracking and auditing processes, data-driven decision-making, and improved compliance to practice guidelines (Alotaibi & Federico, 2017), it also serves as a facilitator of evidence-based practice. However, it has also changed the way people work and communicate, while in some ways influencing expectations for the need for speed and rapid response times, particularly with Generation Y and Generation Z. This means that nursing leaders need to be well-versed in varying communication modalities, and they have to navigate conveying their message in a "timely" manner, a shift from prior generations. Also, because these two newer generations are considered technology-based learners, a leader's development strategies for this group of learners need to encompass a technological aspect (e.g., interactive apps, websites, YouTube videos, podcasts, or infographics) to help ensure that information is delivered according to their preferred learning style (Pearson, 2018). Again, another shift.

In addition to utilizing a more technology-based development approach, leaders need to further adapt their leadership approaches to meet the needs of Generation Y and Generation Z—groups that have notoriously bucked the traditional, command-and-control style of leadership (Post, 2024; Carew International, 2025). Though transformational leadership and authentic leadership yield positive results, today's generations need more. They need leaders who can teach them, leaders who can develop them, leaders who can create a learning environment, leaders who can offer support in a sometimes destabilizing environment, leaders who can help them move up in the organization, and leaders that utilize a coaching style of leadership to coach them (Albert et al., 2022; Sherman, n.d.). This need for new leadership is not restricted to healthcare systems; it is equally applicable across the nursing disciplines (e.g., those in higher education). So, how do leaders adapt to meet this new need? They can start by refocusing their mindset, conversation style, and feedback delivery.

Coaching Mindset

Some leaders may believe they lead with a coaching mindset, but research shows that leaders are still "directing" as opposed to coaching (Sherman, 2023). One of the core competencies put forth by the ICF requires coaches to embody a coaching mindset. They further explain that coaches should maintain an open, client-centered, curious mindset. Additionally, ICF denotes eight needed elements to meet this competency (2020, p. 2). The skilled coach:

1. Acknowledges that clients are responsible for their own choices
2. Engages in ongoing learning and development as a coach
3. Develops an ongoing reflective practice to enhance one's coaching
4. Remains aware of and open to the influence of context and culture on self and others
5. Uses awareness of self and one's intuition to benefit clients
6. Develops and maintains the ability to regulate one's emotions
7. Mentally and emotionally prepares for sessions
8. Seeks help from outside sources when necessary

Though the above eight elements embodying a coaching mindset are a required expectation for ICF certified coaches, these elements are threaded into almost every step or recommendation for building a coaching mindset that can be found on the internet—in blogs, articles, ChatGPT output, and other scholarly sources(Kee et al., 2010; Polemis, 2023; Rindlisbacher, 2020; Sherman, 2023). A compilation of some of the recommendations include:

- Reflects on past experiences
- Leadership reflects on self

- Advocates continued education and development
- Recognizes individuals are resourceful
- Creates a safe environment
- Actively listens and poses thoughtful questions
- Presents clear expectations
- Sets goals
- Respects the client's autonomy
- Reacts nonjudgmentally

Learning Checkpoint

Use the table below to review the coaching mindset elements. In each "How" column, indicate how you could integrate the elements into your current leadership practice.

ICF Coaching Mindset	How	Coaching Mindset (other)	How
Acknowledges that clients are responsible for their own choices		Reflects on past experiences	
Engages in ongoing learning and development as a coach		Leadership reflects on self	
Develops an ongoing reflective practice to enhance one's coaching		Advocates continued education and development	
Remains aware of and open to the influence of context and culture on self and others		Recognizes individuals are resourceful	
Uses awareness of self and one's intuition to benefit clients		Creates a safe environment	
Develops and maintains the ability to regulate one's emotions		Actively listens and poses thoughtful questions	
Mentally and emotionally prepares for sessions		Presents clear expectations	
Seeks help from outside sources when necessary		Sets goals	
		Respects the client's autonomy	
		Reacts nonjudgmentally	

Learning Checkpoint

Consider the coaching mindset elements you need to integrate into your leadership practice. Which one is the most important?

Coaching Conversations

Reflecting back, Chapters 1 and 2 defined and discussed coaching as a leadership development tool aimed toward helping the client generate solutions to their own problems or challenges, establishing pathways to new opportunities, fostering current skills, and developing new skills. Remember, coaching is largely comprised of posing skillful, powerful, open-ended questions in an intellectually stimulating dialogue exchange. Therefore, coaching can really be threaded into almost *any* conversation. Because formal, hours-long conversations are unnecessary, coaching is a feasible implementation for busy leaders, reducing the overused mantra "not enough time" (Albert et al., 2022, p. 520; Sherman, n.d.).

When leaders engage in coaching conversations, almost any topic applies. Some topics can include behavioral issues, leadership behaviors, professional development needs, motivation, engagement, teamwork, emotional intelligence, delegation efforts, communication delivery, response to feedback, change agility, etc. This, of course, is not an all-encompassing list, but it shows that coaching conversations can be wide-ranging.

The purpose of this text is not to certify nurse leaders as executive coaches; there are specialized programs for that. Rather, this text aims to provide leaders with the tools they need to utilize coaching as a means of development for their clients. Coaching takes practice and requires authentic delivery. Therefore, the best way to begin to implement the coaching conversation is to practice! To prepare for the coaching conversation, leaders can draft or review a list of stimulating, open-ended questions. Sherman (n.d.) suggests choosing a few go-to questions that are comfortable for you to open the conversation with the client. Example coaching questions can be found at the end of Chapter 1, but Sherman (n.d.) also provides a kick-start question list. The following are some questions Sherman (n.d.) included on her list:

- What's on your mind?
- What is the real challenge here for you?
- What matters most to you in your practice?
- What talents do you know you have but are not using?
- How can you do more of the work you love?
- What actions do you need to take but are avoiding?
- What are the best sources of feedback for you to measure your progress?

While there are kick-start questions to consider as Sherman (n.d.) notes, there are also questions and behaviors that leaders should *avoid*. Though some of these were threaded into earlier chapters, it is worth reconsidering the following behaviors:

- Asking more than one question at a time (also known as stacking)
- Asking closed-ended questions
- Asking leading or directive questions (e.g., you like this new development program, right?)
- Oversharing your experience(s)
- Offering advice when it was not requested
- Being preoccupied (e.g., checking phone, email, watch, etc.)
- Over celebrating milestones (small celebrations are ok)
- Not acknowledging emotions
- Fixating on emotions
- Not allowing enough time for the client to think and respond to the question posed (yes, a few moments of silence are ok!)
- Not measuring success
- Putting too much pressure on yourself (e.g., constantly thinking about the next question you are going to ask your client instead of letting the process flow)

Also, it is important to understand that coaching is not feedback and feedback is not coaching. However, the coach can utilize a feedback–coaching approach to promote learning and development and enhance performance.

Feedback Type

As giving and receiving feedback is an essential element of leadership, it is necessary to understand feedback type or categorization and feedback delivery. There are between four and 10 types of feedback, depending on the source consulted. Let's review some of the feedback type technology "hits" that are front and center when the phrase "types of feedback" is searched.

The Leading Effectively staff (2023) list four types of feedback, including (a) directive, (b) contingency, (c) attribution, and (d) impact. In brief, and according the Leading Effectively staff (2023), directive refers to telling someone what or how to do something; contingency provides someone with a future consequence (e.g., if you continue to treat people this way, no one will want to work with you); attribution feedback occurs when labels are added to the feedback (e.g., excellent speaker, strong writer, skillful communicator); lastly, impact feedback is largely performance oriented.

The Center for Instructional Technology and Training (n.d.) at the University of Florida neatly categorizes feedback as being either (a) formal, (b) informal, (c) summative, or (d) formative. Like any good academic institution, they also provide a best practice list for applying such feedback, and of course, web links to additional information. According to the university, formal feedback occurs in a consistent fashion (e.g., grading); informal feedback can occur at random (e.g., through conversation or impromptu class discussion); summative feedback is more like the final assessment of a course or topic; and formative is provided when opportunities for growth can be demonstrated (e.g., resubmitting an assignment).

The rapid rise of artificial intelligence (AI) has allowed the generation of ChatGPT 3.5 responses to the question what are the different types of feedback? Below are the automated responses:

- **Positive feedback:** This type of feedback focuses on highlighting and reinforcing positive behavior, performance, or outcomes. It's meant to encourage and motivate individuals by acknowledging their strengths and achievements.
- **Constructive feedback:** Also known as developmental feedback, this type aims to provide specific suggestions for improvement. It focuses on areas where the individual can grow, offering actionable advice and pointing out areas that need attention.
- **Negative feedback:** While it sounds critical, negative feedback isn't necessarily bad. It addresses issues or areas for improvement but should be delivered in a constructive manner, emphasizing solutions rather than just highlighting problems.
- **Formative feedback:** This feedback is given during the process or while a task is ongoing. It's aimed at guiding and shaping the ongoing work, allowing for adjustments and improvements as the work progresses.
- **Summative feedback:** This type of feedback is given at the end of a process or task. It evaluates the final outcome, providing an overall assessment of the performance without necessarily offering guidance for future improvements.
- **360-Degree feedback:** This feedback involves input from multiple sources, including peers, supervisors, subordinates, and sometimes even external stakeholders. It provides a comprehensive view of an individual's performance from various perspectives.
- **Written feedback:** Feedback conveyed through written means, such as emails, reports, or notes. This can include detailed explanations, examples, and suggestions for improvement.
- **Verbal feedback:** Given orally, either in person or over the phone, verbal feedback can be immediate, allowing for real-time discussion and clarification.
- **Continuous feedback:** Instead of waiting for specific review periods, continuous feedback involves ongoing communication and dialogue between parties. It's a more fluid approach to addressing performance and improvements as they arise.

Utilization of AI comes with its own pros and cons, but for busy clinicians, the ease of access and timely return of information is an attractive feature. Though healthcare systems provide resource support, such as librarians or shared governance councils that can complete a scholarly search for any topic of interest, using these resources takes time. During a time-sensitive situation or even during a moment of curiosity, accessing sources that return instant results are the most realistic option. However, I would be remiss if I didn't state that AI, in its current state, **does not and should not** replace traditional, scholarly research or evidence-based practice recommendations because the content produced is not always accurate.

Feedback Delivery

Having a grasp on the types of feedback is a crucial first step in understanding how to deliver it. Now that types of feedback have been reviewed, feedback delivery can be discussed. Because some of the aforementioned types of feedback (e.g., written) are self-explanatory in the delivery, this section will focus on the types that require one-to-one conversation. This snapshot of feedback delivery guides leaders to more of a coaching-based conversation. Additionally, it is worth mentioning that feedback *and* coaching are critical to fostering healthcare providers' growth, development, and competency (Atkinson et al., 2022).

Logemann (2023), part of the Forbes Business Council, outlines a broad, six-step approach for feedback delivery. In this feedback delivery process, the first step requires leaders to have a one-to-one in-person meeting (if possible) with clear, direct discussion points. Once the meeting has commenced, leaders provide specific details regarding the situation at hand; ideally, these conversations should occur in close proximity to the situation to allow prompt reflection and provide real-time feedback. Leaders should focus on the situation or action *not* the person, and they should provide problem-solving examples to stimulate solution generation. Perhaps the most important element of this particular approach is *making the feedback conversational*, which includes engaging clients in the process and asking stimulating questions. Lastly, the leader should be open to the notion that they may be greeted with criticism during the conversation; however, composure, empathy, and professionalism should never wane.

For leaders who like a simpler, clearer, more directive framework, the Center for Creative Leadership (2022) situation—behavior—impact (SBI) model for feedback is both easy to remember and easy to implement. The SBI model or framework focuses on presenting the situation, using clear descriptors and evidence of the situation; delivering the feedback/describing the behavior(s) in a judgment-free tone; and describing the results of the behavior. To enhance the delivery of this model, the leader can *add an element of inquiry* to further acknowledge or explore the client's viewpoint regarding the situation. Sherman (2019) notes that exploration should occur with open-ended questions, which can provide an opportunity for coaching.

The stop—keep doing—start (SKS) model, developed by Phil Daniels is another three-step approach that is relatively easy to employ (Mind Tools Content Team, 2023b). This model is question oriented and comprises the following three specific questions:

1. What should you (the person in question) stop doing?
2. What should you (the person in question) keep doing?
3. What should you (the person in questions) start doing?

This method, is action-focused, requires the person in question to think deeper, and allows leaders to engage in stimulating feedback in a short amount of time (Mind Tools Content Team, 2023b). With the *open-ended questioning* within this model, leaders are shifting toward a coaching style.

The CEDAR feedback model follows more of a *coaching approach*. This model allows the recipient of the feedback to take the lead in the conversation (Mind Tools Content Team, 2023a). The CEDAR acronym is written out as follows:

- **C**ontext
- **E**xamples
- **D**iagnosis
- **A**ction
- **R**eview

In the first step, the leader applies "context" meaning, he or she sets the stage for feedback by reinforcing the notion that the client's performance matters in multiple aspects (e.g., personally, departmentally, and organizationally). Then the leader can provide examples of situations or tasks that need to be discussed. Importantly, following the presentation of the situation or task, the leader should invite the client to share their point of view or opinion of the topic at hand. The leader can initiate this by asking open-ended questions (e.g., How do you see this?). Once the leader has gained insight into the client's perspective, an action plan can be developed. Again, this step should be initiated with open-ended questions (e.g., what actions do you need to take to resolve this?). Lastly, is review. Just as with any typical leadership conversation, follow-up is essential to sustaining success. For this reason, leaders employing this framework should ensure follow-up meetings are in place.

Each of these feedback models intertwines itself with coaching and is a great first step in making the transition into leader–coach. Leaders need to utilize a coaching approach to their conversations and everyday leadership practices to meet the needs of today's workforce. To ensure departmental or organizational success, leaders must fundamentally shift the way in which they interact and converse with their employees—that is, they need to assume a coaching mindset (Ibarra & Scouler, 2019; Sherman, 2023).

How to Apply Coaching in the Nurse Leader Role

Nurse leaders, irrespective of the setting, work under a large span of control, wear many hats, and are pressured to maximize engagement and productivity, while fostering a healthy work environment—with Generation Y and Generation Z bringing a new perspective—and creating a culture of teaching, learning, growth and development. In addition, nurses lead a multigenerational workforce, directly contribute to positive organizational outcomes, and prepare for the unseen challenge (Best, 2020; Roussel et al., 2023). Coaching can be quite impactful on all the above, but applying coaching may feel outside of some nurse leaders' wheelhouse, and rightfully so. Nurse leaders are not trained or taught the ins and outs of coaching. Nursing programs, particularly graduate programs with a leadership or administrative focus, have coaching threaded somewhere in an assignment or part of required readings, but there is no in-depth conversation or teaching surrounding coaching in nursing. With the shift to competency-based education in nursing (which pairs beautifully with coaching), along with the continued calls for a paradigm shift in leadership, nursing education needs to do more to help current and emerging leaders develop their coaching skill set.

More needs done on the organizational level as well. Unfortunately, many organizations do not provide nurse leaders with professional development opportunities related to coaching or offer nurse leaders coaches, unless they are part of the executive leadership team. This is a missed opportunity. And although *some* organizations provide a high-level overview of coaching as part of the leadership summits or as a learning opportunity for those interested, it's not enough to move the needle for leadership change.

Nevertheless, leaders can learn more about coaching through self-guided education or certification programs (see Chapter 10 for more information on these programs). By applying some of the principles and practices presented thus far in this text, nurse leaders can integrate coaching into their everyday practices. They can then begin to:

- Strengthen trust and rapport with their direct reports and team members
- Adapt leadership styles to meet the needs of the unit, team, or direct report
- Reframe leadership conversations to encompass a coaching style that includes the following:
    - setting clear goals
    - asking open-ended, powerful questions (individually—don't complicate the conversation)
    - embracing silence and long pauses
    - establishing metrics

- evaluating progress
- providing feedback and development when necessary
- acknowledging success

Though this list appears to include features easily implemented, it does take practice to shift from a traditional feedback style conversation to a coaching conversation. Remember, coaching conversations do not need to be formal, hour-long conversations.

Where and When to Have a Coaching Conversation

Depending on what type of leadership role one assumes (e.g., executive, director, or manager), having frequent one-to-one meetings with direct reports can be quite challenging, or even unrealistic if the span of control is too large or one-to-one meetings are an unfamiliar practice within the leader's respective setting. However, some type of leader–direct report meeting can be conducted. Interestingly, results from the AONL Foundation's nursing leadership insight study (2022) contained data from over 2,300 nursing leaders across the nation and established that nearly 80% of nursing leadership tasks encompassed meeting with direct reports and colleagues. Of these respondents, 50% reported this was the task that provided them the most joy.

Importantly, leaders can engage in a coaching conversation almost anywhere—during morning/evening huddles or morning/evening staff greetings, leadership rounds, team meetings, and of course the one-to-one meeting (Sherman, n.d.). These conversations can be quick interactions, lasting anywhere from 5 to 15 minutes, which can also be viewed as micro-coaching sessions. Micro-coaching sessions are focused, brief bite-size conversations that can occur in real time, within the normal workflow (Clark, 2020). Similar to traditional coaching, micro-coaching aims to improve behavior, performance, satisfaction, and stimulate learning (Spangler, 2023). Micro-coaching is also goal-oriented and action driven, just like traditional coaching. Given the short duration of the sessions, micro-coaching can occur more frequently, as opposed to traditional coaching, which occurs in a more structured and sometimes lengthy process. Additionally, in today's workforce where immediate feedback and response is expected, this approach is effective and time efficient. However, though micro-coaching is beneficial and more appealing and feasible for leadership application, there is a time and place for traditional coaching.

When Not to Coach

Though coaching can be immensely impactful, it cannot replace some of the directiveness that is required from those in leadership roles. In academia, some faculty and students are not coachable. The same is true for nursing staff; some individuals just do not want to be coached. As discussed in previous chapters, those who are not coachable will not reap the benefits of coaching, so these individuals need a more directive approach. There are also circumstances where coaching may not be appropriate, including:

- When past or current emotional turmoil is impacting the workplace (counseling or therapy should be explored for the client in these circumstances)
- When a client lacks the knowledge base or skill set (e.g., new nurse that has never been exposed to placement of an external ventricular drain or a junior faculty who has never created an online course)
- When an urgent situation requires direct instruction
- When expectations are being communicated
- When dealing with complex performance management issues (though coaching can be utilized *after* feedback has been given)

Coaching does not replace the need for management; rather, it serves as a tool for managers to improve performance, productivity, confidence, satisfaction, and teamwork, while building a coaching culture (Richardson et al., 2023; Rodine, 2021).

Summary

Nursing leaders are tasked with numerous challenges, irrespective of their setting. With the evolution of technology, workforce demographics, and fluctuating financial health, leaders need tools and resources to lead in a complex environment. Leaders can positively impact their organizations by applying the principles of coaching in everyday leadership practices. However, applying these principles and shifting to a coaching style of leadership takes practice.

Resources

Case Example

Calista, a seasoned faculty member in academia who has chaired various committees and served in interim leadership roles throughout her 12-year tenure, transitioned into a program director position within the last 15 months. Her duties are similar to what they would be at other universities and include budgeting and fiscal management, teaching, managing and overseeing faculty and their productivity, development, performance, completing research and service responsibilities, maintaining communication with accrediting bodies, leading all accreditation efforts, evaluating curriculum, formulating/strengthening community partnership for nursing advisory boards, engaging in institutional advancement efforts, and collaborating with academic, student life, and human resources departments for current and future department/student initiatives. Calista states these newfound responsibilities have "been quite a transition" but she believes she has adapted well and has been successful over the last 15 months. However, after reviewing her most recent 360-assessments, she was both "surprised and disappointed," especially because she had a strong relationship with colleagues before moving into the director role and felt they would be supportive of her in the new role.

Nevertheless, Calista carefully reads the feedback and begins to make note of comments that require attention. In doing this, Calista notices several areas where improvement is needed. She has prioritized two prominent themes for action:

- singular, dated approach to leadership
- feedback provided in a one-directional way with little opportunity for conversation

As part of Calista's action plan, she has requested an executive coach (partially paid with her professional development funds) to help her develop better leadership practices.

Reflecting on the information in this chapter and previous chapters, how would you as the executive coach perform the following actions:

- Conduct the initial meeting
- Decide/integrate assessments (including the 360s)
- Review assessments/debrief results
- Establish client's goals
- Coach (what framework *could* you use—e.g., GROW, CLEAR, etc.)
- Integrate metric evaluation

Midway through the coaching engagement, you suggest that Calista send out another round of 360 evaluations. Results indicate that Calista has been applying a more transformational approach to leadership, which is a great finding. However, there are still comments indicating that Calista is struggling with delivering feedback (she is still utilizing a one-way approach feedback delivery). What questions might you pose to Calista to challenge her to *explore* and *apply* a more coaching-directed framework for delivering feedback? List at least five.

Understanding When to Apply the Coaching Conversation—and When Not To

Coaching conversations can occur with almost any leadership conversation. List 7 to 10 opportunities where you, as the leader-coach, can apply a coaching conversation.

1. ______________________________
2. ______________________________

3. ______________________________
4. ______________________________
5. ______________________________
6. ______________________________
7. ______________________________

For each of the examples noted above, pose one question to start the conversation surrounding that topic.

1. ______________________________
2. ______________________________
3. ______________________________
4. ______________________________
5. ______________________________
6. ______________________________
7. ______________________________

Discussion/Reflection Question: Coaching Culture

Review the following resources:

https://www.ccl.org/articles/leading-effectively-articles/instill-coaching-culture/

https://journals.lww.com/jphmp/fulltext/2021/05000/building_a_coaching_culture_the_roles_of_coaches,.19.aspx

https://coachingfederation.org/app/uploads/2019/01/CaseStudy_HSE.pdf

After reviewing the resources, discuss how you, as a leader, can begin to create a culture of coaching in your workplace. Be sure to include discussion on stakeholder buy-in and resources needed to begin this process.

Real-World Application

Coaching skills evolve with practice. With this in mind, find three individuals to coach. They may choose any work-related or leadership topic. The session does not need to be long—aim for 15 to 20 minutes. Be sure to identify the topic and set the goal for the session before you begin to coach. Be sure to ask only open-ended questions. Once you have completed the session, debrief the conversation. Ask them to provide information on what was helpful and what was not. What questions stimulated them to think deeper, and what things need to be improved for future conversations? Keep a log of your feedback for future use.

References

Albert, N., Pappas, S., Porter-O'Grady, T., & Malloch, K. (2022). *Quantum leadership: Creating sustainable value in health care* (6th ed). Jones and Bartlett.

Alotaibi, Y. K., & Federico, F. (2017). The impact of health information technology on patient safety. *Saudi Medical Journal*, *38*(12), 1173–1180. https://doi.org/10.15537/smj.2017.12.20631

American Organization for Nursing Leadership Foundation. (2022). Longitudinal nursing leadership insight survey part four: Nurse leaders top challenges and areas for needed support, July 2020-August 2022. (www.aonl.org)

Atkinson, A., Watling, C. J., & Brand, P. L. P. (2022). Feedback and coaching. *European Journal of Pediatrics*, *181*(2), 441–446. https://doi.org/10.1007/s00431-021-04118-8

Best, K. (2020). *Power bases: A great tool for the leadership coach*. International Coaching Federation. https://coachingfederation.org/blog/power-bases-leadership-tool

Carew International. (2025). *Leading gen Z: Adapting your leadership style for a new generation*. https://www.carew.com/leading-gen-z/#:~:text=The%20Gen%20Z%20generation%20is,need%20for%20reskilling%20are%20prevalent.

Center for Creative Leadership. (2022). *Use situation-behavior-impact (SBI) to understand intent*. https://www.ccl.org/articles/leading-effectively-articles/closing-the-gap-between-intent-vs-impact-sbii/

Center for Instructional Technology and Training. (n.d.). *Types of feedback*. University of Florida. https://citt.ufl.edu/resources/assessing-student-learning/providing-effective-feedback/types-of-feedback/

Clark, T. (2020, October 6). The importance of micro-coaching: A pandemic survival skill. *Forbes*. https://www.forbes.com/sites/timothyclark/2020/10/06/how-to-create-your-teams-virtual-vibe-with-microcoaching-a-pandemic-survival-skill/?sh=65a8b1a41a4c

Ibarra, H., & Scouler, A. (2019). The leader as coach. *Harvard Business Review*. https://hbr.org/2019/11/the-leader-as-coach

International Coaching Federation (ICF). (2020). *ICF core competencies*. https://coachingfederation.org/credentials-and-standards/core-competencies

Kee, K., Anderson, K., Dearing, V., Harris, E., & Shuster, F. (2010). The coach leader mindset: the cognitive shift. In *RESULTS coaching: The new essential for school leaders* (1st ed., pp. 9–22). Corwin Press, https://doi.org/10.4135/9781452219646; https://us.sagepub.com/sites/default/files/upm-assets/36204_book_item_36204.pdf

Leading Effectively Staff. (2023, May 19). *How to give the most effective feedback*. Center for Creative Leadership. https://www.ccl.org/articles/leading-effectively-articles/review-time-how-to-give-different-types-of-feedback/

Logemann, R. (2023, February 9). The art of delivering constructive feedback. *Forbes*. https://www.forbes.com/sites/forbesbusinesscouncil/2023/02/09/the-art-of-delivering-constructive-feedback/?sh=1598981c77a3

Mind Tools Content Team. (2023a). *Cedar Framework Model*. Mind Tools. https://www.mindtools.com/a3951oq/the-cedar-feedback-model

Mind Tools Content Team. (2023b). *Stop—keep doing—start*. Mind Tools. https://www.mindtools.com/agu1o7v/stop-keep-doing-start

Pearson. (2018, May 24). *What do generation z and millennials expect from technology in education?* https://www.pearson.com/en-us/higher-education/insights-and-events/teaching-and-learning-blog/2018/05/generation-z-millennials-expect-technology-education.html

Polemis, J. (2023). *The coaching mindset*. Coaching for Leadership. https://wp.nyu.edu/coaching/mindset/

Post, J. (2024, January 22). *What do millennials want in a modern leader?* Business.com. https://www.business.com/articles/leadership-styles-millennials/

Richardson, C., Wicking, K., Biedermann, N., & Langtree, T. (2023). Coaching in nursing: An integrative literature review. *Nursing Open*, *10*(10), 6635–6649. https://doi.org/10.1002/nop2.1925

Rindlisbacher, D. (2020). Coach mindset: Preparing leaders to create a climate of trust and value. *Nursing Administration Quarterly*, *44*(3), 251–256. DOI: 10.1097/NAQ.0000000000000430

Rodine, R. (2021, March 9). *5 reasons coaching for nurse leaders is imperative*. Inspire Nurse Leaders. https://inspirenurseleaders.com/5-reasons-coaching-for-nurse-leaders-is-imperative/

Roussel, L., Thomas, P. L., & Harris, J. L. (2023). *Management and leadership for nurse administrators* (9th ed.). Jones & Bartlett.

Sherman, R. (n.d.). *Fueling RN professional growth.* AONL. https://www.aonl.org/publications/voice/fueling-rn-professional-growth-steps-adopt-leader-coach-mindset

Sherman, Rose. (2019). The art of giving feedback. *American Journal of Nursing, 119*(9), 64–68. DOI: 10.1097/01.NAJ.0000580292.79525.d2

Sherman, R. (2023, March 9). *Developing a coaching mindset.* EmergingRNLeader. https://emergingrnleader.com/developing-a-coaching-mindset/

Spangler, D. (2023, April 19). *How to use micro-coaching for teacher PD.* eSchool News. https://www.eschoolnews.com/educational-leadership/2023/04/19/how-to-use-micro-coaching-for-teacher-pd/

CHAPTER 5

COACHING TO BUILD AND SUSTAIN CAPITAL

This chapter will include ways that nurse leaders can build and sustain capital. This chapter will build upon prominent texts in graduate-level nursing courses as it pertains to maximizing capital; however, the application of coaching to build *human* and *psychological capital* will be the focus.

Chapter Objectives

1. Examine the impact of human capital
2. Explore how coaching can build human capital
3. Examine the constructs of psychological capital
4. Analyze how coaching can build psychological capital

Types of Capital

Capital is a type of resource or asset that can generate value, revenue, or influence well-being (Avey et al., 2011; CFI Team, 2024b). There are various types of capital, including financial, social, physical, intellectual, human, and psychological (the latter two will be described in further details in their own subsequent sections). The following bullet points provide a brief summary of each type of capital:

- **Financial capital:** This refers to monetary assets used to facilitate business operations (e.g., provide services, sales, or marketing), investments, and acquisitions (Ross, 2023).
- **Social capital:** Social capital refers to "the presence of networks, relationships, shared norms, and trust among individuals, teams, and business leaders—[it] is the glue that holds organizations together" (Lauricella et al., 2022, para. 1).
- **Physical capital:** Physical capital refers to the tangible assets that contribute to the production of goods and services. Common examples include operating equipment (e.g., machinery), infrastructure, and technology (CFI Team, 2024b).
- **Intellectual capital:** As stated by CFI Team (2024a, para 1), intellectual capital "refers to the value of a company's collective knowledge

and resources that can provide it with some form of economic benefit." Intellectual capital can be further categorized into three branches: relational, structural, and human.

- **Human capital:** Human capital represents the knowledge, skills, expertise, experience, and abilities held by individuals (Kenton, 2023).
- **Psychological capital:** Psychological Capital (PsyCap) is a set of internal resources, consisting of hope, efficacy, resiliency, and optimism (Luthans et al., 2015).

Effective management and investment in these different forms of capital are essential for sustaining growth, innovation, and overall success—whether in business, society, individual, or professional development. Importantly, when the aforementioned types of capital are fostered, it can positively impact economic growth (e.g., business expansion, new job opportunities), entrepreneurship, innovation, and workplace culture, to name a few (Nuryanto et al., 2020; Ribaj & Mexhuani, 2021). Thus, each type, or a combination of capital, plays a significant role in economic, social, professional, and/or organizational development.

Human Capital

Human capital is a resource that can impact both the micro and macro level of the organization. It drives both performance and productivity (Aman-Ullah et al., 2022; Nickolas, 2023) and is arguably one of the most important resources an organization has (Madgavkar et al., 2022). Because human capital encompasses one's knowledge, skills, expertise, experience, and abilities (Kenton, 2023), it can and should be developed. It should be viewed as an asset (World Economic Forum, 2020). As such, leaders should advocate for their organizations to do the following:

- Make resources available for access to educational initiatives (e.g., conference to keep up to date with workplace trends and best practices, etc.)
- Offer intriguing learning and skill development opportunities for staff (e.g., workshops, skill sessions, or training programs, etc.)
- Provide work-related experience opportunities (e.g., shadowing for those interested in leadership, or participation in leadership summits, or introduction of leadership opportunities through committee work or entry-level roles, such as charge nurse)
- Invest in employees' physical and mental well-being (e.g., workplace stress management programs)
- Create a workplace that is welcoming to *all* persons and communities and provides equal access to opportunities for advancement
- Offer a variety of incentives (e.g., opportunities for additional shifts, coursework overload, paid time off, memberships, meaningful recognition, catered lunches, gift cards, etc.)

- As a leader, participate in leadership development training; access internal or external coaches to build better leadership practices
- Provide coaching to help employees reach their full potential

While these may seem like commonsense initiatives, oftentimes organizations fall short in one or more areas. Thus, it is important for leaders to advocate and ensure employees have equal opportunity for development. Every development opportunity has the potential to lend a hand in the maximization of human capital.

Coaching Culture and Human Capital

Previous chapters discussed the foundation and benefits of coaching, so it should be no surprise that coaching can be used as a tool for building human capital. Coaching can be applied to enhance individuals' skills, capabilities, and overall performance. This, in turn, can bolster confidence, engagement, perceptions of leadership and organizational support, and positively impact the culture of the organization (Albert et al., 2022; Roussel et al., 2023).

More specifically, a strengths-based coaching approach (a positive psychology, solutions-based approach) can be of added value when aiming to build or leverage human capital. As the name implies, strengths-based coaching aims to assess the strengths and talents of an individual (Deweese, 2017). This strengths-based approach is grounded in traditional foundations of coaching (e.g., active listening, client accountability, strategy/action planning). To apply a strengths-based coaching approach, leaders should do the following:

- **Conduct strengths assessments**
    - This can be done formally with tools like the CliftonStrengths to identify employees' top strengths, or informally by seeking informal feedback from colleagues or other supervisors.

- **Create individual development plans**
    - Similar to traditional coaching, leaders should develop personalized coaching plans that build on individual strengths and align with organizational goals.

- **Align roles with strengths**
    - Place employees in roles and projects where they can utilize their strengths.

Leaders must be cautious *not* to do the following (McQuillen, 2021):

- Avoid addressing profound areas of weakness
- Over focus on creating a "well-rounded" employee

- Create situations where employees believe they can avoid responsibilities in any area of weakness (e.g., if the weakness is public speaking, the employee should not avoid presenting or hosting department meetings if it is a job expectation)

Though leaders can influence change when they use a strengths-based coaching approach (or coaching in general), it cannot be sustained without the cultivation of a coaching culture. As a leader, you might be asking *how* can we get to a place where employees across the disciplines value coaching and have access to coaching? *How* can an organization who is managing financial constraints provide managers and leaders with advanced training or certification for coaching? These are all great questions, and the answer is through culture change.

Leaders looking to soft launch a coaching culture can thoughtfully and consistently employ coaching conversations, demonstrate the value of coaching to senior or executive leaders, and equip other stakeholders with coaching conversations skills (Funck, 2023). In essence, "better culture starts with better conversation" (Funck, 2023, para 1.). For those looking to hard launch, time, dedication, persistence, collaboration, innovation, and layering (or a step-by-step approach) are fundamental to the success of the culture change. A culture change plan can be helpful to better manage this launch. The Wharton School, the business school of the Ivy League University of Pennsylvania, introduced a Nano Tool, a leadership tool that can be learned and implemented in 15 minutes.

In brief, this five-step process first requires leaders to quantitatively measure the current culture and values. This can be done utilizing employee surveys and organizational assessments. Next, leaders align culture, strategy, and structure. Then they can engage the stakeholders to assist in designing and building the desired change process or culture. Step four encompasses various and copious communication—and demonstration of the change. Lastly, managing the response is a critical to the success and sustainability of the initiative. Of note, emotional intelligence is an absolute necessity in times of change; it influences leadership effectiveness. For more information on each step of the nano tool, please view the following site:

https://executiveeducation.wharton.upenn.edu/wp-content/uploads/2018/03/1409-Managing-Culture-Change.pdf

Requirements for a Coaching Culture

During the last decade, the ICF has partnered with the Human Capital Institute (HCI) to study the tenets of a coaching culture, (HCI, 2023, p. 7), which include the following:

1. Employees value coaching
2. Senior executives value coaching

3. Mangers/leaders and/or internal coaches received accredited coaching-specific training
4. Coaching is a fixture in the organization with a dedicated line item in the budget
5. Managers/leaders (and/or internal coach practitioners) spend an above-average amount of their weekly time on coaching activities
6. All employees in the organization have an equal opportunity to receive coaching from a professional coach practitioner

Organizations who perceive their organization to have a strong culture reported their organizations having met at least five of the above elements.

This report can be viewed at the following link:

Other reports, beginning with the 2014 report up to and including the 2023 report, can be viewed at the link below. (There is a small fee to view six studies if you are not a member of ICF.)

https://coachingfederation.org/research/building-a-coaching-culture

Learning Checkpoint

Think about your own organization as you reflect on the tenets of a coaching culture. Are they meeting any of the tenets? If so, which one(s)? If not, where can you advocate for change?

Psychological Capital

Historically, psychology focused on mental illness and inappropriate or dysfunctional behaviors (Luthans & Youssef-Morgan, 2017). However, after decades of disregarding the potential of healthy, successful individuals, Dr. Martin Seligman posed a new call during his American Psychological Association presidential address of 1998 entitled "A Call to Research the Healthy, Happy, and Human Potential of Individuals—A Call for 'Positive Psychology'" (Luthans & Youssef-Morgan, 2017). This new call for positive psychology within the field ignited fierce interest among scholars and practitioners, leading to an exponential increase in research. This, in turn, inspired research in the fields of management and organizational behavior. And management and organizational behavior literature began to emphasize the application of positive psychology in the workplace (Luthans & Youssef-Morgan, 2017).

Interestingly, this development of positive psychology was a relatively new concept for most organizations. Traditionally, organizational research focused on negative factors, namely, burnout, dissatisfaction, ineffective leadership behaviors, and unjust cultures (Luthans & Youssef-Morgan, 2017; Luthans et al., 2015). The hyperfocus on negative factors resulted in lack of research on positive initiatives such as high performers, well-being, and managing the transitions for strategic change and sustainability, to name a few (Luthans & Youssef, 2007; Luthans et al., 2015).

Organizational and behavioral scholars continued their exploration into positive psychology and recognized positive organizational scholarship (POS). POS, an umbrella concept, integrates positive perspectives, approaches, and processes that can enhance workplace performance outcomes (Garza-Wrigley, 2015; Luthans & Youssef-Morgan, 2017; Luthans et al., 2015). Findings from POS research helped structure a more specific concept, positive organizational behavior or (POB), and later PsyCap.

POB can be broadly defined as positive internal human strengths and psychological capacities that can be developed and managed for workplace performance (Luthans, 2002). According to this definition, for something to be considered a psychological capacity, it must be developable and related to performance outcomes (Garza-Wrigley, 2015; Luthans et al., 2015). These positive psychological capacities, which include hope, efficacy, resiliency, and optimism, became known as driving factors for creating competitive markets in business, medicine, and even academic settings.

More specifically, this newfound focus on psychological capacities became the foundation for the higher construct of PsyCap (Luthans & Youssef, 2007; Luthans et al., 2015). PsyCap can be defined as having the ability to create and achieve professional and personal goals (hope), confidence to embrace and complete challenging tasks (efficacy), ability to bounce back from challenging setbacks (resiliency), and hopefulness about present and future success (optimism) (Luthans & Youssef, 2007).

Comprehending the definitions and constructs of PsyCap individually aids in understanding PsyCap as a higher order construct. PsyCap hope was drawn from Snyder's theory of hope, which can be defined as a positive emotional state that enables an individual to draw from agency or willpower to create goals and determination or waypower to achieve goals (Snyder et al., 2002). Importantly, Luthans et al. (2015) states:

> One's willpower and determination motivates the search for new pathways, while creativity, innovation, and resourcefulness involved in developing pathways in turn ignites one's energy and sense of control, which when taken together result in an upward spiral of hope. (p. 83)

In relation to nursing, professional goals are generated through creativity, innovation, and resourcefulness. These goals can range from earning an advanced degree or certification (staff nurse), revising course or curricula (educators), to creating interprofessional work teams, community partnerships, and bolstering the pipeline of future leaders.

Next, PsyCap efficacy is defined as "one's belief about his or her ability to mobilize the motivation, cognitive resources, and courses of action necessary to execute a specific action within a given context" (Stajkovic & Luthans, 1998 as cited by Luthans, 2015, p. 30). Efficacy, deeply rooted in Bandura's social cognitive theory, contains five specific cognitive processes that are critical to efficacy (Luthans, et al., 2015). These five processes include (a) symbolizing, (b) forethought, (c) observation, (d) self-regulation, and (e) self-reflection.

Symbolizing refers to one's ability to create a mental image, develop a process or decision-making model from that image, and use the imagery as a guide for action. *Forethought* allows one to plan for both actions and consequences based on previous experiences, namely, successes and failures. *Observation* derives from observing behaviors or responses that yielded positive responses learned from those in one's social network (e.g., colleagues, management). *Self-regulation* requires one to set high standards and specific goals to achieve a desired performance. Constant assessment helps to ensure that the desired standards and goals will be met. Lastly, *self-reflection*, which may be the most crucial to efficacy, requires one to look back on previous actions, successes, and failures and extract situations or experiences that can be modified for the future. Importantly, self-reflection can enhance self-regulation, self-awareness, and self-development, which are vital for professional growth. Professional growth can bolster a nurse's confidence in their role, which in turn can promote retention, productivity, and job satisfaction (American Association of Critical Care Nurses [AACN], 2024; Parsons, 2022).

Following efficacy, is PsyCap resiliency. "Resiliency" has many definitions; however, PsyCap resiliency focuses on the positive organizational perspective and can be defined as "the capacity to rebound or bounce back from adversity, conflict, failure, or even positive events, progress, and increased responsibility" (Luthans 2002 as cited by Luthans et al., 2015, p. 145). More specifically, this definition supports the use of adversity as a launching pad for personal growth and development (Luthans et al., 2015). Understanding baseline resiliency can assist leaders in building their employees' resiliency through assessments and trainings.

Lastly, PsyCap optimism is viewed from a global tendency, meaning that one can form positive expectations about life in general. With an explanatory or attributional style, optimism enables one to attribute positively experienced events to personal, permanent, and pervasive causes (Luthans et al., 2015). The fundamental process underlying optimistic style entails one's self-assessment of "response-outcome independence." This means that when one feels in control, the result is a feeling of "immunization" against feelings of helplessness or pessimism, which in turn enables one to fight for a future they wish to see and experience (Luthans et al., 2015). In nursing, optimism assists in navigating complex health system partnerships, mentoring new nurses or faculty, or partnering with interprofessional teams to engage in innovative research initiatives that will generate nationwide recognition and truly advance the science of nursing.

While each construct within PsyCap can be individually developed to foster growth in that specific construct, each construct should be nurtured to promote higher PsyCap as a whole. Higher PsyCap has also been linked to lower employee cynicism, reduced absenteeism, higher organizational citizenship behaviors, and positive interpersonal behaviors (Center for Creative Leadership, 2021; Luthans et al., 2015; Mcdaid, 2020). High PsyCap can also lead to a stronger, healthier, and well-connected workforce (Mcdaid, 2020; Singh, 2023). These critical factors increase work engagement and professional development initiatives (Boamah & Laschinger, 2014).

Psychological Capital and Workplace Behaviors

Workplace behaviors can have implications for organizations—both positive and negative. Organizational citizenship behaviors (OCB) yield positive results. These behaviors occur when an individual welcomes tasks and responsibilities outside of their contractual obligation that support either the individual or the macro-level organization (Avey et al., 2011; Harper, 2015; Luthans et al., 2015). Individuals who display OCB also have higher levels of PsyCap and often report increased job satisfaction, productivity, well-being, and reduced stress, burnout, and turnover intention (Avey et al., 2011; Flinkman et la., 2023; Garza-Wrigley, 2015; Giraldez-Hayes, 2021; Luthans & Youssef, 2007; Luthans, Avolio et al., 2013; Luthans et al., 2015; Singh, 2023).

Counterproductive work behaviors (CWB), on the other hand, are loosely defined as negative behaviors that impede the well-being of employees and the organization as a whole (Avey et al., 2011). Landmark findings from Spector and Fox (2002) suggest that workplace stress is the primary contributor to CWB. Interestingly, individuals with lower levels of PsyCap tend to exhibit CWB as a result of reduced adaptive capabilities to stress and decreased resiliency and hope (Avey et al., 2011). Unfortunately, these maladaptive behaviors and reduced psychological capacities (resiliency and hope) can lead to burnout—a syndrome characterized by feelings of exhaustion, failure, and pessimism (Koutsimani et al., 2019) that can lead to psychological distress. According to the results of a 2020 survey, over 60% of nurses reported feeling burnout (American Nurses association [ANA], 2024). Furthermore, nursing burnout can negatively impact performance outcomes (An et al., 2020).

PsyCap Development and Coaching

McCoy and Smith (2023, para. 8) state that "PsyCap can be thought of as a fuel that supports the pursuit of whatever target or outcome an organization cares most about ... it is development jet fuel." Much like everything else,

PsyCap can be developed via traditional learning modalities (e.g., classroom learning) or through relatively short web-based interventions (Carter & Youssef-Morgan, 2022; Luthans et al., 2008). In addition, recent literature has determined that micro-coaching programs have positively impacted—and sustained—PsyCap post coaching (Corbu et al., 2021). Leaders/manager who utilize a coaching approach "can maximize each component of PsyCap ... by leveraging their role as an additional support to help [staff] problem solve, chart new paths in the face of resistance, accurately appraise their own situations, and practice good coping strategies" (McCoy & Smith, 2023, para. 12).

Each element of PsyCap can also be developed through micro-coaching with blended development opportunities. Corbu et al. (2021) replicated a micro-coaching intervention by Palaez et al. (2020). The program occurred over 5 weeks and followed the GROW/RE-GROW framework. An outline of the program is depicted in Table 5.1 below.

TABLE 5.1 **Corbu et al. (2021) Micro-Coaching Intervention Plan**

Session	Main purpose	Activities/tasks	Homework
1	Connecting and sharing. Pre-assessment results: feedback and reflection. Goal setting. Workbook delivery.	Welcome: coach's presentation and objectives, structure and internal rules of the program; Icebreaker: participants' self-presentation through symbols; Positive psychology inputs; Presentation of the variables assessed and delivery of the results; Goal setting using SMART+ technique: role-playing in pair.	Brief survey to think about the gap between current and desired situation (i.e., How do you define success in your life at this moment? When are you at your best? What are your personal strengths?)
2	Process development following the GROW model: GOAL setting (SMART+), examine the REALITY, explore OPTIONS, and establish the WILL.	Review Session 1: potential areas uncovered (SMART+ goal). **Reality:** identifying and reflecting about personal strengths and weaknesses (symbol identification, strengths map, SWOT analysis). **Options:** brainstorming and analysis of advantages and disadvantages. **Action plan:** detailed description regarding the what, why, when, how, and who questions.	"Timeline" exercise: steps to follow for the action plan. Start the action plan.

(Continued)

TABLE 5.1 **Corbu et al. (2021) Micro-Coaching Intervention Plan (*Continued*)**

Session	Main purpose	Activities/tasks	Homework
3	Follow-up the action plan:	Review Session 2: contents and doubts. Activity: "Time line" adapted to the action plan. Reflection about the achievements so far and future actions. Activity: (written and visualized) "The Best Possible Self" exercise. Process overview	Practice and follow the plan.
4	Closing, review, and reflection	Review Session 3: topics, action plan, and doubts. Coaches' feedback on the process, and coaches' performance.	

SMART, Specific, Measurable, Achievable, Realistic, Time-bound; +, Positive; SWOT, Strengths, Weaknesses, Opportunities, Threats.

Another approach to building PsyCap through coaching is by incorporating a stepwise approach. van Zyl et al. (2020) conducted a systematic review on positive psychological coaching and produced a five-phase model to facilitate professional growth and development. This five-phase model (p. 3) includes the following:

Step 1: Creating the relationship
Step 2: Strength profiling and feedback
Step 3: Developing an ideal vision
Step 4: Goal setting, strategizing, and execution based on strengths
Step 5: Concluding relationship and recontracting

This model is similar to other coaching models described in Chapter 2, whereby the coach explores the problem, establishes equal footing, assesses the situation, creates goals, coaches, and measures/evaluates success. It also overlaps with Corbu et al.'s (2021) micro-coaching intervention plan depicted in Table 5.1 above. However, goal creation and pathway identification (Step 4) should not be rushed. In fact, leaders should spend as much time as needed on developing the willpower (goal creation) and waypower (pathway) for their direct reports. This includes utilizing a goal-making framework, such as SMART, creating an inventory of obstacles, and establishing subgoals and multiple pathways for achieving the goal (Luthans et al., 2013).

For example, if an employee's goal is to submit a manuscript for publication by the end of the year, the leader working with that employee should help make this goal more specific, perhaps suggesting a manuscript title (e.g., *"Staff Nurses Perceptions of Their Leaders Approach to Coaching"*), a suitable journal (e.g., *Journal of Nursing Administration*) and a feasible submission date (e.g., by July 20XX). The leader should also inquire about obstacles to meeting this goal and how that impacts the time frame or goal in general (e.g., will the employee have time for writing the manuscript with her current workload?). If the employee's big-picture goal is to disseminate the findings, the leader should have the employee draft multiple pathways for achieving this (e.g., add other journals, submit for podium or poster presentations, etc.). In short, leaders should always ensure employees have concrete endpoints to measure success, as well as identifying and preparing for obstacles and interruptions along the pathway to achieving the goal. This way, employees can prepare multiple avenues for achieving success.

Psychological Capital for Nursing and Nursing Leadership Development

Leadership is a critical element for nursing growth and development and is supported by large organizations such as the National Academy of Medicine (NAM), National League for Nursing (NLN), Sigma, and the AONL. These organizations advocate, promote, and encourage leadership development for clinical and academic nurses. Nurses are expected to yield leadership attributes that could be enhanced through self-development, personal self-reflection, and coaching (Keaton 2021; Singh & Haynes, 2020). As mentioned earlier, PsyCap is the "jet fuel" for development (McCoy & Smith, 2023).

What do we know about PsyCap and leadership development, and why should we foster it? Empirical research on PsyCap as an indicator for seeking leadership development is still in its infancy. But one study worth mentioning was published in 2018 by Pitichat et al., researchers adapted the original definition of PsyCap to include more specific leadership verbiage, resulting in leadership development (LD) PsyCap. LD PsyCap can be defined as:

> having confidence (efficacy) to take on and put in the necessary effort to succeed at challenging leader development tasks; making a positive attribution (optimism) about succeeding now and in the future in terms of developing as a leader; persevering toward leader development goals and, when necessary, redirecting paths to goals (hope) in order to succeed; and when beset by problems and adversity, sustaining and bouncing back and even beyond (resilience) to attain success at leader development (Pitichat et al., 2018, p. 49).

Pitichat et al. (2018) identified four environmental constructs that impact self-leadership development, including (a) learning climate, (b) organizational support, (c) social support, and (d) workload. These constructs were utilized to detail the cause and effect or presumed relationship to support their research on the newly coined concept of LD PsyCap. In brief, learning climate refers to the fact that organizations prioritizing an environment supportive of learning are better suited to facilitate employees' current and future learning and developmental processes (Pitichat et al., 2018). Organizational support occurs when employees perceive senior leadership as supportive and considerate of their professional needs (Pitichat et al., 2018). Social support, while similar to organizational support, differs slightly, including the support employees perceive from their colleagues (Pitichat et al., 2018). Lastly, workload defines the amount of work required in one's role (Pitichat et al., 2018).

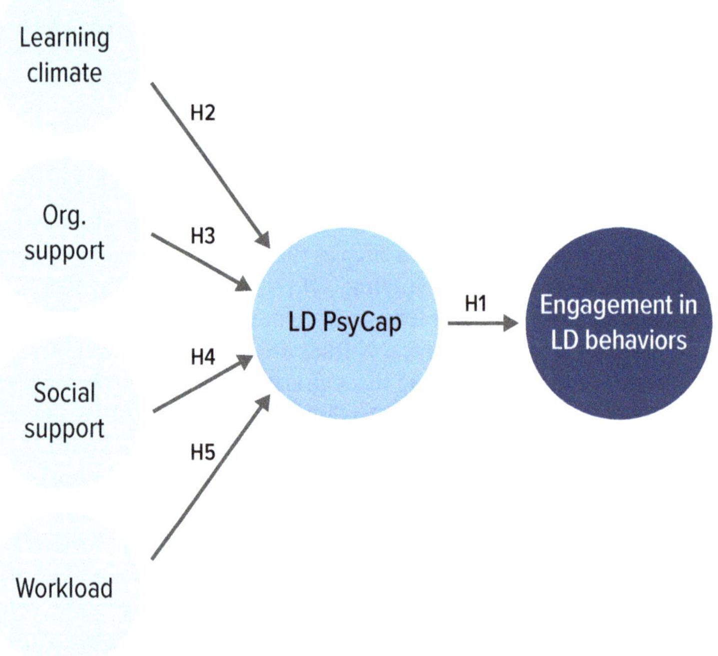

FIGURE 5.1 Pitichat et al. (2018) Model

Source: Thiraput Pitichat, Rebecca J. Reichard, Amber Kea-Edwards, Eric Middleton and Steven M. Norman, "Model," *Psychological Capital for Leader Development*. Copyright © 2018 by Oxford University Press.

Following the establishment of LD PsyCap and the constructs of the work environment, the researchers recruited 120 leaders across the United States who previously participated in trainings or assessments given by a regional consulting firm. Findings suggested that LD PsyCap not only predicted leader development behaviors, but it also mediated the relationship between the four components of the work environment. Given that PsyCap is developable, it may be advantageous for senior or executive leadership to explore development opportunities for their employees, especially those who verbalize intent to seek formal leadership roles. This is especially important given the repeated call for nurses to engage in leadership development, with the most recent call coming from *The Future of Nursing 2020–2030: Charting a Path to Achieve Health Equity* (NAM, 2021). This report continues to emphasize the need for constant engagement in leadership development to assist nurses across the discipline in moving forward personally, professionally, and within their respective communities.

More importantly, nurses who choose to engage in leadership training can learn to adapt and model necessary leadership behaviors, further promote the organization's mission and vision, foster a culture of diversity, equity, and inclusion, create action learning assignments, such as a leadership and/or management simulation. They demonstrate effective decision-making in an uncertain clinical environment and indirectly or directly influence peer or follower PsyCap (Chen et al., 2017; Center for Creative Leadership, 2021; Kouzes & Posner, 2017; Onley, 2019; Singh & Haynes, 2020).

Summary

This chapter provided an overview of the varying types of capital, including financial, social, physical, and intellectual, emphasizing human and psychological. Human capital and PsyCap are essential elements for employee and organizational growth and development. Leaders have the tools and resources to foster both, but coaching is the key for sustainability.

Resources

Discussion/Reflection Question

In your department, you have an employee who feels her strengths are not being leveraged appropriately. As a leader, you know a strengths-based coaching approach would work best with this employee. Describe what your next steps might look like for the employee, including the coaching plan.

Critical Reflection

- Which component of PsyCap (hope, self-efficacy, resilience, or optimism) do you believe is the most critical to develop in today's workforce, and why?
- What challenges might managers face when trying to implement a strengths-based coaching strategy? How can they overcome these obstacles?
- Can focusing on strengths inadvertently lead to blind spots in professional development?

PsyCap Development Plan: Goal Creation and Pathway Identification

In Table 5.1, Corbu et al. (2021) depicted that during Session 2 of their PsyCap micro-coaching session, time is spent on goal development (this would relate to the element of hope within PsyCap). In order to help direct reports or peers with professional goals, leaders should be able to draft their own layered goals and prioritize accordingly. However, sometimes, leaders create vague, overarching goals for themselves, which makes measurement and evaluation challenging. Using a SMART framework (or other framework), draft three goals: (a) professional, (b) personal, and (c) community. Include an inventory of potential obstacles and at least two alternate pathways for achieving the goals.

References

Albert, N., Pappas, S., Porter-O'Grady, T., & Malloch, K. (2022). *Quantum leadership: Creating sustainable value in health care* (6th ed). Jones and Bartlett.

Aman-Ullah, A., Mehmood, W., Amin, S., & Abbas, Y. A. (2022). Human capital and organizational performance: A moderation study through innovative leadership. *Journal of Innovation & Knowledge,* (7)4, p. 1–9. https://doi.org/10.1016/j.jik.2022.100261.

American Association of Critical Care Nurses. (2024, September 4). *Nurse retention strategies and resources.* Nurse Retention Strategies and Resources

American Nurses Association. (2024). *What is nurse burnout? How to prevent it.* Nurse Burnout: What Is It & How to Prevent It | ANA

An, M., Shin, E. S., Choi, Y. M., Lee, Y., Hwang, Y. Y., & Kim, M. (2020). Positive psychological capital mediates the association between burnout and nursing outcomes among hospital nurses. *International Journal of Environmental Research and Public Health, 17*(16), 5988. https://doi.org/10.3390/ijerph17165988

Avey, J. B., Reichard, R. J., Luthans, F., & Mhatre, K. H. (2011). Meta-analysis of the impact of positive psychological capital on employee attitudes, behaviors, and performance. *Human Resource Development Quarterly, 22*(2), 127–152. https://doi:10.1002/hrdq.20070

Boamah, S., & Laschinger, H. (2014). Engaging new nurses: The role of psychological capital and workplace empowerment. *Journal of Research in Nursing, 20*(4), 265–277. https://doi.org/10.1177/1744987114527302

Carter, J., & Youssef-Morgan, C. (2022). Psychological capital development effectiveness of face-to-face, online, and micro-learning interventions. *Education and Information Technologies, 27,* p. 6553–6575. https://doi.org/10.1007/s10639-021-10824-5

Center for Creative Leadership. (2021). *4 reasons to invest in leadership development.* https://www.ccl.org/articles/leading-effectively-articles/why-leadership-development-is-important-4-reasons-to-invest/

CFI Team. (2024a). *Intellectual capital.* CFI. https://corporatefinanceinstitute.com/resources/valuation/intellectual-capital/

CFI Team. (2024b). *Physical capital.* CFI. https://corporatefinanceinstitute.com/resources/economics/physical-capital/

Chen, Q., Zhonglin, W., Yurou, K., Niu, J., & Hau, K. T. (2017). Influence of leaders' psychological capital on their followers: Multilevel mediation effect of organizational identification. *Frontiers in Psychology, 8*, 1–19. https://doi.10.3389/fpsyg.2017.01776

Corbu, A., Pelaez Zuberbuhler, M. J., & Salanova, M. (2021). Positive psychology micro coaching intervention: Effects on psychological capital and goal-related self-efficacy. *Frontiers in Psychology, 12*, 1–14. https://doi.org/10.3389/fpsyg.2021.566293

Deweese, C. (2017, February 15). *How to make your coaching truly strengths-based.* Gallup. https://www.gallup.com/cliftonstrengths/en/250382/coaching-truly-strengths-based.aspx

Flinkman, M., Coco, K., Rudman, A., & Leino-Kilpi, H. (2023). Registered nurses' psychological capital: A scoping review. *International Journal of Nursing Practice, 29*(5), e13183. https://doi.org/10.1111/ijn.13183

Funck, F. (2023, January 9). *How to instill a coaching culture.* Center for Creative Leadership. https://www.ccl.org/articles/leading-effectively-articles/instill-coaching-culture/

Garza-Wrigley, S.D. (2015). *Who are you and what do you do? Psychological Capital and leadership: A study of the differences in Psychological Capital of leaders in various careers.* [Unpublished doctoral dissertation]. Our Lady of the Lake University.

Giraldez-Hayes, A. (2021). Coaching to develop psychological capital to support change. In W.-A. Smith, I. Boniwell, & S. Green (Eds.), *Positive psychology coaching in the workplace.* Springer, Cham. https://doi.org/10.1007/978-3-030-79952-6_14

Harper, P. J. (2015). Exploring forms of organizational citizenship behaviors (OCB): Antecedents and outcomes. *Journal of Management and Marketing Research, 18*, 1–16. https://www.aabri.com/manuscripts/142119.pdf

Human Capital Institute. (2023). *Defining new coaching cultures.* www.hci.org

Keaton, M. (2021). *National League for Nursing announces selections for 2021 leadership institute.* https://www.nln.org/newsroom/news-releases/news-release/2021/01/21/nln-announces-selections-for-2021-leadership-institute

Kenton, W. (2023, December 18). *Human capital definition: Types, examples, and relationship to the economy.* Investopedia. https://www.investopedia.com/terms/h/humancapital.asp

Koutsimani, P., Montgomery, A., & Georganta, K. (2019). The relationship between burnout, depression, and anxiety: A systematic review and meta-analysis. *Frontiers in Psychology, 10*, 284. https://doi.org/10.3389/fpsyg.2019.00284

Kouzes, J., & Posner, B. (2017). *The leadership challenge: How to make extraordinary things happen in organizations* (6th ed.). Jossey-Bass.

Lauricella, T., Parsons, J., Schaninger, B., & Weddle, B. (2022, August 2). *Network effects: How to rebuild social capital and improve corporate performance.* McKinsey & Company. https://www.mckinsey.com/capabilities/people-and-organizational-performance/our-insights/network-effects-how-to-rebuild-social-capital-and-improve-corporate-performance

Luthans, F. (2002). Positive organizational behavior: Developing and managing psychological strengths. *Academy of Management Executive, 16*(1), 57–52. https://doi.org/10.5465/ame.2002.6640181

Luthans, F., Avey, J., & Patera, J. (2008). Experimental analysis of a web-based training intervention to develop positive psychological capital. *Management Department Faculty Publications,* 135. http://digitalcommons.unl.edu/managementfacpub/135

Luthans, F., & Youssef, C. M. (2007). Emerging positive organizational behavior. *Journal of Management, 33*(3), 321–349. https://doi.org/10.1177/0149206307300814

Luthans, F., & Youssef-Morgan, C. (2017). Psychological capital: An evidence based positive approach. *Annual Review of Organizational Psychology and Organizational Behavior, 4,* 339–346. https://doi.org/10.1146/annurevorgpsych-032516-113324

Luthans, F., Youssef-Morgan, C., & Avolio, B. (2015). *Psychological capital and beyond.* Oxford University Press.

Luthans, F., Avolio, B. J., & Avey, J. B. (2013). *Trainer's guide for developing psychological capital.* Mind Garden. https://www.mindgarden.com/psychological-capital-questionnaire/209-psycap-trainers-guide.html

Madgavkar, A., Schaninger, B., Smit, S., Woetzel, L., Samandari, H., Carlin, J., & Chockalingam, K. (2022, June 2). *Human capital at work: The value of experience.* McKinsey & Company. https://www.mckinsey.com/capabilities/people-and organizational-performance/our-insights/human-capital-at-work-the-value-of-experience

McCoy, K., & Smith, D. (2023). *How coaching creates better leaders: Exploring the role of psychological capital.* CCL. https://cclinnovation.org/news-posts/how_coaching_creates_better_leaders_exploring_the_role_of_psychological_capital/#:~:text=Put%20another%20way%2C%20effective%20coaching,transformative%20outcomes%20down%20the%20line.&text=PsyCap%20can%20be%20thought%20of,an%20organization%20cares%20most%20about.

Mcdaid, E. (2020). *In difficult times, look for a HERO.* Leaders Edge. https://www.leadersedge.com/brokerageops/indifficult-times-look-for-a-hero

McQuillen, B. (2021, July 14). *How strengths-based coaching optimizes human capital.* Ignite. https://www.ignitehcm.com/blog/guide-to-strengths-based-coaching

National Academy of Sciences, National Academy of Engineering, and National Academy of Medicine (NAM). (2021). *The future of nursing 2020–2030: Charting a path to achieve health equity.*

Nickolas, S. (2023, October 28). *What is the relationship between human capital and economic growth?* Investopedia. https://www.investopedia.com/ask/answers/032415/what-relationship-between-human-capital-and-economic-growth.asp#:~:text=Human%20capital%20refers%20to%20the,can%20lead%20to%20icreased%20productivity

Nuryanto, U. W., N., Dajamil M., Sutawidjaya, A. H., & Saluy, A. B. (2020, May). The impact of social capital and organizational culture on improving organizational performance. *International Review of Management and Marketing, 10*(3), p. 93–100.

Onley, D. (2019). *How leaders can make better decisions.* SHRM. https://www.shrm.org/hrtoday/news/hr-magazine/fall2019/pages/how-leaders-can-make-better-decisions.aspx

Peláez, M. J., Coo, C., and Salanova, M. (2020). Facilitating work engagement and performance through strengths-based micro-coaching: A controlled trial study. *J. Happiness Stud.* 21, 1265–1284. doi: 10.1007/s10902-019-00127-5

Parsons, L. (2022, August, 23). *Why is professional development important?* Harvard Division of Continuing Education. Why is Professional Development Important? - Professional & Executive Development | Harvard DCE

Pitichat, T., Reichard, R. J., Kea-Edwards, A., Middleton, E., & Norman, S. M. (2018). Psychological capital for leader development. *Journal of Leadership & Organizational Studies, 25*(1), 47–62. https://doi.org/10.1177/1548051817719232

Ribaj, A., & Mexhuani, F. (2021). The impact of savings on economic growth in a developing country (the case of Kosovo). *Journal of Innovation and Entrepreneurship, 10*, 1. https://doi.org/10.1186/s13731-020-00140-6

Ross, S. (2023). *Financial capital vs. economic capital: What's the difference?* Investopedia. https://www.investopedia.com/ask/answers/031715/what-difference-between-financial-capital-and-economic-capital.asp

Singh, A. (2023). Psychological capital among nursing faculty: Implications for practice. *Nurse Educator*, 1–6. https://doi.org/10.1097/NNE.0000000000001430

Singh, A., & Haynes, M. (2020). The challenges of COVID-19 in nursing education: The time for faculty leadership training is now. *Nurse Education in Practice, 47*, https://doi.org/10.1016/j.nepr.2020.102831

Snyder, C. R., Rand, K. L., & Sigmon, D. R. (2002). Hope theory: A member of the positive psychology family. In C. R. Snyder & S. J. Lopez (Eds.), *Handbook of positive psychology* (pp. 257–276). Oxford University Press.

Spector, P. E., & Fox, S. (2002). An emotion-centered model of voluntary work behavior: Some parallels between counterproductive work behavior and organizational citizenship behavior. *Human Resource Management Review, 12*(2), 269–292. https://doi.org/10.1016/S1053-4822(02)00049-9

van Zyl, L. E., Roll, L. C., Stander, M. W., & Richter, S., (2020, May 5). Positive psychological coaching definitions and models: A systematic literature review. *Frontiers in Psychology, 11*, 793. https://doi.org/10.3389/fpsyg.2020.00793

Wharton Aresty Institute of Executive Education. (2014, September). *Five steps to managing culture change.* https://executiveeducation.wharton.upenn.edu/thought-leadership/wharton-at-work/2014/09/managing-culture-change/

World Economic Forum. (2020, August 19). *Human capital as an asset: An accounting framework to reset the value of talent in the new world of work.* https://www.weforum.org/publications/human-capital-as-an-asset-an-accounting-framework-to-reset-the-value-of-talent-in-the-new-world-of-work/

Zhu, Y., Tsai, C.-Y., Wang, Y., & Guo, Z. (2023). Does Leader-Follower PsyCap Congruence Cultivate Change-Related Outcomes? A Supervisor-Subordinate Fit Perspective. *Journal of Leadership & Organizational Studies, 30*(1), 25–39. https://doi.org/10.1177/15480518221132037

CHAPTER 6

COACHING TO BUILD LEADERSHIP BEHAVIORS

This chapter will describe ways nurse leaders can apply coaching to build their direct reports' leadership behaviors, specifically transformational, authentic, and situational.

Chapter Objectives

1. Examine transformational leadership
2. Examine authentic leadership
3. Examine situational leadership
4. Explore the application of coaching to build leadership practice

Transformational Leadership

Transformational leadership is a leadership style that focuses on inspiring and motivating followers to achieve exceptional performance and personal growth. This approach emphasizes the leader's ability to create a vision for the organization or team, to communicate that vision effectively, and to empower and support individuals to contribute toward achieving it. Transformational leadership has been associated with numerous benefits, including higher employee satisfaction, increased motivation, engagement, and organizational citizenship behaviors, improved performance, productivity, and greater organizational culture (Khan et al., 2020; Kurnat et al., 2017; Steinmann et al., 2018; Ystaas et al., 2023). It is particularly well-suited to dynamic and challenging environments where innovation, adaptability, and collaboration are essential for success—contributing to its prominence.

Importantly, the notion that transformational leadership only applies to those in formal administrative roles should be dismissed. As discussed in previous chapters, the title of leader is not reserved for those who hold a formal administrative title; in fact, leaders are threaded throughout every layer of an organization. Each individual's or team's leadership behaviors/practices has the potential to influence the organization culture (Bass & Avolio, 1994), which then impacts satisfaction, performance, productivity, intent to stay, and more (Abane et al., 2022; Iskamto, 2023).

Nurses have undoubtedly been introduced to transformational leadership (in its broadest sense) either through workplace conversations with their leaders (especially those employed in a Magnet designated hospital) or through marketing initiatives promoting transformational leadership as a core organizational or expected behavior. Additionally, for those pursuing advanced nursing degrees, nursing leadership textbooks provide highlights of transformational leadership. Here are a few excerpts from leadership textbooks on transformational leadership:

> Transformational leadership has been defined as a superior form of leadership that occurs when leaders bring awareness to the shared or common desires of leaders and followers. This awareness, commitment, and acceptance of the purposes of the mission, of the group or organization are motivating factors followers embrace as they look beyond self-interest and embrace change for the good of the group (Harris et al., 2022, p. 370).

> Transformational leaders are energetic, compassionate, and enthusiastic. They have the ability to provide a vision, motivate, and inspire others (Melnyk & Fineout-Overholt, 2019, p. 335).

> Transformational leadership is defined as a state in which leaders and followers find meaning and purpose in their work and grow and develop as a result of their relationship (Barker et al., 2006 as cited in Melnyk & Raderstorf, 2021, p. 16).

Though these excerpts display the big picture of transformational leadership, discussion on the seminal work and concepts are often omitted, with the exception of Broome and Marshall's (2021) text entitled *Transformational Leadership in Nursing*, which takes a deeper dive into these concepts. Nevertheless, understanding the aforementioned is critical for nurse leaders who wish to better position themselves in their coaching role.

Background

Pulitzer Prize winning biographer, political scientist, and leadership scholar James McGregor Burns is considered the founding father of transformational leadership, bringing attention to the concept in the 1970s, which makes it one of the oldest methodological and psychological approaches in leadership (Alessa, 2021). During Burn's time as presidential biographer and informal advisor to United States presidents, he observed transformational leadership as a process of "leaders and followers raising each other to high levels of morality and motivation" (Mind Tools Content Team, 2024a, para 1). He argued that transformational leaders inspire and motivate followers to transcend their own self-interests and work toward a collective vision or higher purpose.

While Burns is rightfully credited with uncovering transformational leadership, Bernard Bass's work has been instrumental in shaping and popularizing it as a distinct leadership approach throughout research and practice. Specifically, Bass identified four behaviors and characteristics associated with transformational leadership, including (a) charisma or idealized influence/charisma, (b) inspirational motivation, (c) intellectual stimulation, and (d) individualized consideration. These are known as Bass's four I's of transformational leadership (Figure 6.1). We will consider each of these individually.

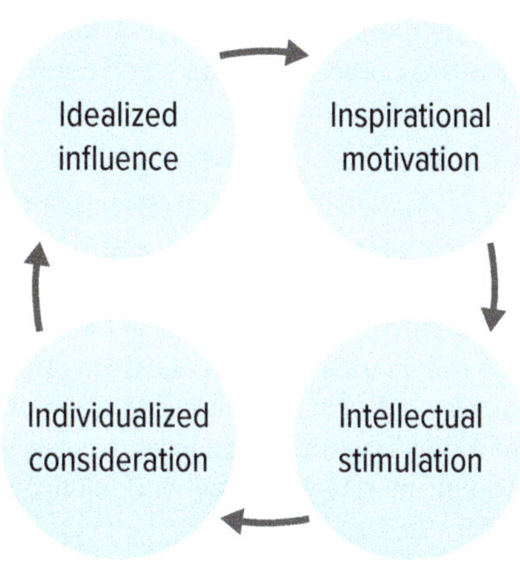

FIGURE 6.1 Bass's 4I's of TL

Idealized Influence

Idealized influence or charisma is one's ability to provide a sense of mission, instill pride, and gain respect and trust (Bass, 1990, p. 22). Charismatic leaders are role models who display qualities of transparency, authenticity, and accountability to earn their follower's confidence (Broome & Marshall 2021; Ystaas et al., 2023). They put others needs before their own and lead by example (Quality Improvement Center for Workforce Development, 2022).

Inspirational Motivation

Inspirational motivation occurs when one can enthusiastically communicate expectations, use symbols to focus efforts, or express important purposes in simple ways (Bass, 1990). It enables leaders to create captivating speeches, paint a vivid, positive big picture, and instill a sense of meaning and optimism, which is the foundation for creating an inspiring vision for the future (Ystaas et al., 2023). They encourage creativity, innovation, and a commitment to excellence. They also inspire a shared vision among their followers and colleagues.

Intellectual Stimulation

Intellectual stimulation promotes intelligence, rationality, and careful problem-solving (Bass, 1990). Intellectual stimulation is critical for challenging boundaries and moving beyond the status quo. Leaders not only ask their followers to think outside the box, but they also nurture independent thinking during the process (Broome & Marshall, 2021). They promote a culture of learning, experimentation, and continuous improvement.

Individualized Consideration

Individualized consideration refers to the degree to which a leader recognizes, understands, values, and supports their followers or team members' individualities. They understand when to incorporate different strategies, *including coaching*, mentorship, hands-on support, empathy, and active listening to foster the growth of others (Broome & Marshall, 2021). Leaders who display individualized consideration proudly acknowledge the contributions of individuals and participate in celebrating the wins, fostering a supportive, and ultimately, healthier work environment.

Building on Transformational Leadership Approach

Kouzes and Posner, best known for their work on exemplary leadership, particularly their book *The Leadership Challenge*, continued to build upon transformational leadership. Through extensive research and survey data, they introduced a transformational leadership model—the exemplary leader, which encompassed five practices of exemplary leadership (Deeb, 2023). These practices included (a) modeling the way, (b) inspiring a shared vision, (c) challenging the process, (d) enabling others to act, and (e) encouraging the heart (Figure 6.2). These five practices serve as a model for leaders to

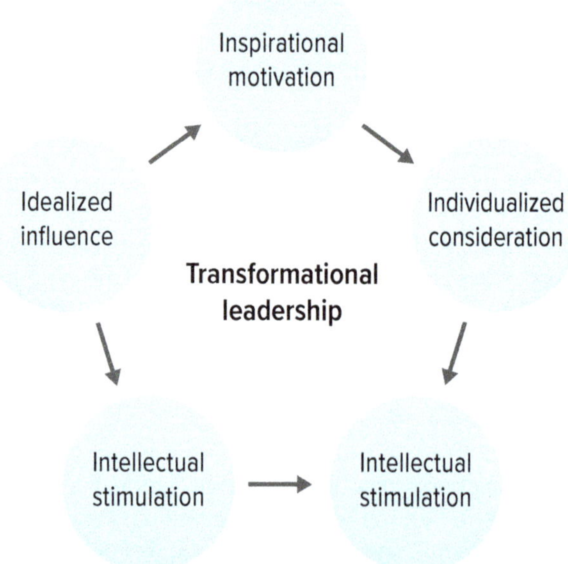

FIGURE 6.2 Five Practices of Exemplary Leadership

inspire and empower others, build strong relationships, and achieve extraordinary results. Kouzes and Posner argue that anyone, regardless of position or level of authority, can develop and strengthen their leadership skills by focusing on these core principles to become exemplary leaders.

Model the Way

Exemplary leaders set the example by aligning their actions with shared values and guiding principles. They establish standards of excellence and lead by example, demonstrating integrity, authenticity, and consistency in their behavior.

Kouzes and Posner (2017) identified two main elements for this practice: (a) clarifying values and (b) setting the example. According to their research, to be an exemplary leader, one must have a complete grasp on their morales, values, beliefs, and ideals and they must be transparent and authentic communicators. These individuals are the ones who "walk the talk" and capitalize on the "we" versus the "I."

Inspire a Shared Vision

Kouzes and Posner (2017) state that the leader must:

- Know where their passion lies
- Reflect on past and current experiences to uncover what is meaningful
- Be able to stop, observe, and process important points of conversation and social discontents
- Spend more time thinking about the future vs. current state
- Actively listen to what others deem important
- Involve others in creating a shared vision

Once these six components are met, the exemplary leader can inspire and mobilize others, envision possibilities, and share a vision that resonates with every member of their team.

Challenge the Process

Exemplary leaders think outside of the box; they embrace challenges and they are not afraid of failure. They experiment, take risks, and encourage others to think creatively and embrace change (Kouzes and Posner, 2017). They encourage innovation and growth by seeking experiences that will challenge the status quo and by continually asking "what's new, what's next, and what's better?" (Kouzes & Posner, 2017, p. 168).

Enable Others to Act

To enable others to contribute and succeed, the exemplary leader must foster collaboration and empowerment (Kouzes & Posner, 2017). They build trust and support and strengthen others through influence, development, and increasing self-determination (Kouzes & Posner, 2017). To do this, Kouzes and Posner (2017) state the leader must do the following:

1. Always be trustworthy
2. Take the time to *really* know team members
3. Be empathetic
4. Actively listen
5. Collaborate in a way that shows others they are interdependent of another
6. Encourage and coordinate face-to-face interactions to foster collegiality

Encourage the Heart

Exemplary leaders recognize and celebrate the contributions of others (Kouzes & Posner, 2017). They bring out the very best in their team. They show appreciation, express gratitude, and celebrate milestones, values, victories, and achievements—fundamental elements for creating a positive and supportive work environment. Exemplary leaders do not engage in predictable, impersonal contributions; rather, they truly exercise personalized, meaningful recognition of each of their team members.

Authentic Leadership

Authentic leadership is a leadership approach that emphasizes genuineness, honesty, transparency, optimism, self-awareness, and moral character (Melnyk & Raderstorf, 2021). Authentic leaders strive to align their actions with their values and beliefs, build trusting relationships with others, and inspire followers through authenticity and integrity. Authentic leadership leads to organizational effectiveness, increased performance, and individual flourishing (AlMazrouei, 2023; Kleynhans et al., 2022).

Background

Bill George, former chairman of Medtronic, executive fellow at Harvard Business School, and former professor at Harvard, is credited with introducing authentic leadership with the 2004 publication of his book entitled *Authentic Leadership: Rediscovering the Secrets to Creating Lasting Value*. This book yielded a wealth of knowledge for current and emerging leaders and also propelled other scholars to further explore this area of leadership.

Some scholars who expanded on authentic leadership included leadership author Peter Northouse, who has helped to further define and clarify the concept within the broader field of leadership studies. Bruce Avolio, a professor, has conducted research on authentic leadership and its impact on organizational outcomes. Fred Luthans, founding father of PsyCap, further explored the relationship between authentic leadership and positive PsyCap, highlighting the importance of authenticity in promoting employee well-being and organizational effectiveness. Professor Michael Brown has focused on the ethical dimensions of authentic leadership and the importance of authenticity within this realm. Lastly, and from the discipline of nursing is Rosanne Raso. Rosanne has contributed to the expansion of authentic leadership throughout the nursing disciplines as speaker, vice president and chief nursing officer, editor-in-chief, nursing manager, and most notably exploring its impact in the work environment. The four dimensions or components of authentic leadership encompass (a) self-awareness, (b) relational transparency, (c) balanced processing, and (d) moral perspective (Figure 6.3), which we will consider next.

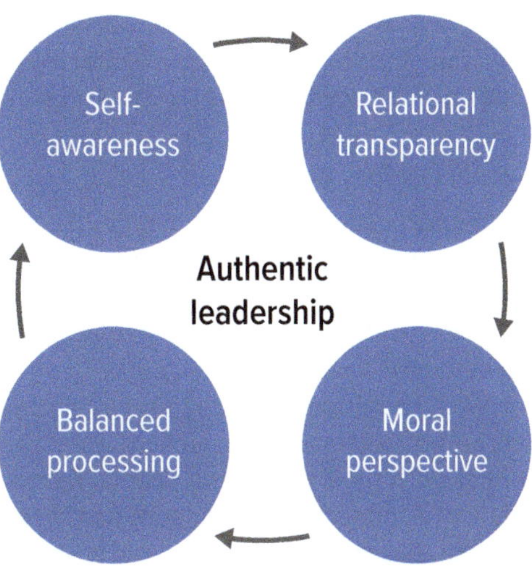

FIGURE 6.3 Authentic Leadership

Self-Awareness

To be truly self-aware, one must have a sound understanding of their strengths, weaknesses, values, and emotions (Riggio, 2014; Lowe, 2021). Authentic leaders are in tune with their inner selves and are aware of how their actions impact others.

Relational Transparency

Authentic leaders build trust through honesty, openness, and integrity. They communicate openly, share information, admit mistakes, and eliminate or mitigate inappropriate or unfavorable situations when necessary (Lowe, 2021). This transparency fosters a sense of trust and respect among followers and open dialogue among the team, which encourages a positive, moral climate in the workplace.

Balanced Processing

Authentic leaders seek out diverse perspectives. They solicit opposing viewpoints to challenge their thought process and carefully consider different viewpoints before making decisions, which demonstrates an unbiased perspective (Riggio, 2014; Lowe, 2021). By engaging in balanced processing or a fair-minded approach, authentic leaders make informed decisions that consider the needs and interests of all stakeholders.

Moral Perspective

Authentic leaders have a strong moral compass and adhere to ethical principles and values. They act with integrity and demonstrate a commitment to doing what is right, even when faced with challenges or pressure to compromise their values. This dimension reflects the importance of ethical leadership in authentic leadership theory.

With these components in mind, authentic leaders are genuine and sincere—both privately and publicly. They practice leadership in a manner that aligns with their values and beliefs, fostering trust among their staff. Their ability to connect with their staff further promotes credibility and trustworthiness. Research shows that trust within the workplace bolsters employees' likelihood of offering ideas and solutions by 23%, contributing to a culture of engagement (Ladika, 2021). This culture of engagement creates awork environment where employees are both valued and respected. Interestingly, respect has been listed as the most important leadership behavior (Rogers, 2018).

In terms of feeling valued, Cande (2022) highlighted the notion that feeling valued at work can lead to better physical and mental health, enhanced satisfaction, increased motivation, and higher levels of engagement. This, in turn, can foster stronger healthier relationships between employees and management. Thus, authenticity is an inspirational motivator for employees across the disciplines.

Additionally, authentic leaders are comfortable with vulnerability and willing to admit their mistakes. This characteristic creates an environment where learning and growth are encouraged, enabling employees to adapt to changing circumstances and bounce back from setbacks more effectively. Authentic leaders, guided by their core values, prioritize ethical considerations in their decision-making process, ensuring that their actions are consistent with principles of fairness, integrity, and responsibility (Menguin, 2024). Overall, authentic leadership fosters a positive organizational culture by enhancing employee engagement, satisfaction, morale, and performance (Baquero, 2023; Duarte et al., 2021; Shick, 2023). Ultimately, authentic leadership contributes to the long-term success and sustainability of the organization at large.

Learning Checkpoint

Think about Bass's four I's and Kouzes and Posner's five practices of exemplary leadership. What areas do you think you excel in? Where do you think you fall short? How can your shortcomings impact your ability to hold impactful coaching conversations?

Situational Leadership

Situational leadership is a leadership model that was developed by Paul Hersey, behavioral scientist and entrepreneur, and Ken Blanchard, management expert and author, in the late 1960s and early 1970s (Wolf, 2022). It suggests that effective leadership varies, depending on the situation and the readiness or maturity of the followers. Situational leadership proposes that leaders should adapt their leadership style based on the specific needs of their team members or followers (Brigden, 2022).

Background

The Hersey-Blanchard situational leadership model was first presented in their *Management of Organizational Behavior: Utilizing Human Resources* book published in 1969. This work has been distributed to over one million individuals during its lifespan. Though this book has undergone several updates (currently in the tenth edition) and continues to build upon Hersey and Blanchard's work, the foundational principles remain. One such principle explains that this model encompasses four distinct leadership styles (The Center for Leadership Studies, 2024), which are as follows:

1. **Telling, directing, or guiding**: In this style, leaders provide specific instructions and closely supervise their team's execution. This approach is designed to generate movement.
2. **Selling, coaching, or explaining**: In this style, leaders provide guidance and support while still maintaining a degree of control. They explain decisions and solicit buy-in from the team.
3. **Participating, collaborating, or facilitating**: In this style, leaders focus on collaborating with followers and facilitating their involvement in decision-making. They provide support and encouragement as needed but aim to enhance task mastery.
4. **Delegating, empowering, or mentoring**: In this style, leaders provide minimal guidance and allow followers to take ownership of the task and to provide insight, suggestions, and improvement strategies.

Additionally, the following four competencies coincide with the above styles (The Center for Leadership Studies, 2024):

1. **Diagnosing** involves the assessment of self (e.g. check and control impulses, thinking before doing) and the readiness of their team members. This competency gives the leader understanding of where each individual is in terms of responsibility and action.
2. **Adapting** leadership style accordingly after diagnosing the readiness of self and team (see above styles). The leader is cognizant of the differing styles needed for each individual within their team.

3. **Communicating** effectively is critical in any leadership position and with any leadership style. Leaders need to not only understand where their own development needs are, but also recognize internal and external factors that could influence the conversation.
4. **Advancing** in situational leadership requires the leader to recognize that organizations are never stagnant and change and innovation are always needed, which supports the notion that both the leader and their team should be ready to investigate and implement strategies that add value to the team and organization.

The above four leadership styles and competencies can assist nursing leadership in the following skills:

- **Optimizing flexibility**: By being flexible in their approach, leaders can effectively address varying levels of readiness, competence, and commitment among their team and provide the needed support in real time.
- **Maximizing effectiveness**: Leaders who can identify the most appropriate style for each situation can maximize their leadership effectiveness and enhance the productivity of their teams.
- **Empowering followers**: Situational leaders embrace delegation to trusted members of their team, increasing employee responsibility and promoting empowerment.
- **Developing talent**: Leaders can determine the readiness of their team members and provide appropriate coaching, and opportunities for growth. This not only helps individuals build competence and confidence over time, but it can also positively influence performance and satisfaction (Pasaribu et al., 2022).
- **Enhancing communication**: By establishing clear expectations, providing relevant feedback, and being receptive to employee feedback, leaders can both promote and maintain a positive working relationship with their team members.
- **Building trust**: Situational leadership builds trust and rapport between leaders and followers. When leaders demonstrate an understanding of their team members' needs and provide appropriate support, it fosters trust, respect, and loyalty within the team.
- **Navigating change**: In times of change or uncertainty, situational leadership provides a framework for leaders to effectively navigate challenges. By assessing the readiness of their team members and adapting their own leadership approach according to the teams needs, leaders can guide their teams through transitions and overcome obstacles.
- **Improving decision-making**: Situational leadership encourages leaders to involve their team members in decision-making processes.

By soliciting input and considering different perspectives, leaders can make more informed decisions that are aligned with the needs and goals of the team.

Overall, situational leadership is important because it helps leaders effectively manage diverse teams, develop talent, foster collaboration, and achieve better outcomes in a variety of organizational contexts. By recognizing the dynamic nature of leadership and adjusting their approach accordingly, leaders can create a positive and productive work environment that promotes growth and success.

This model has various training programs, materials, and tools available to help leaders apply its principles effectively. It's worth noting that "Situational Leadership®" is a registered trademark of The Ken Blanchard Companies. More information on learning solutions or training programs can be viewed here:

https://situational.com/situational-leadership/

Coaching Builds Better Leadership Practices

As we learned from previous chapters, coaching can play a significant role in professional and leadership development through intellectually stimulating conversation, action planning, and evaluation. Using these same fundamental elements, coaching can help foster transformational, authentic leadership, and situational behaviors. Now that principles, behaviors, and competencies of transformational, authentic, and situational leadership styles are understood, coaches can use these elements to build a client's leadership profile based on the client and organizational need.

It is important to reiterate that external coaches will have a more formal coaching process that involves recurring sessions, whereas the leader as coach will utilize a more informal process through recurrent one-to-one coaching conversations, or micro-coaching. Irrespective of the process within one respective organization, it is important to work with the client to tackle the most pressing area first. To determine priority focus areas, the coach should engage in open-ended dialogue and work with the client to determine where growth is desired. During this conversation, the coach can be listing said topics. Once the conversation surrounding focus areas has concluded, the coach and client can rank the most important topics. Ranking can be completed by simply marking "1" as most important and "10" as least important (the ranking scale will depend on the number of topics listed; if there are only six topics, then the last ranked item would be a 6). The table below depicts how coaching can build stronger transformational and authentic leadership behaviors, which can feed into situational leadership.

TABLE 6.1 **Transformational and Authentic Leadership Behaviors**

Focus Area	Application
Self-awareness	Explore the current/emerging leaders strengths and weakness. Through reflective questioning, activities, assessments, and feedback, leaders will gain a deeper understanding of themselves and create a development plan (Peters, n.d.).
Values and motives clarification	Assist the current/emerging leaders in identifying their core values, principles, and motives. By understanding what matters most, they can make decisions and action plans that are consistent with their values (Mind Tools Content Team, 2024b).
Embracing vulnerability	Create a safe space for current/emerging leaders to explore/discuss their vulnerabilities/fears. Through open and honest dialogue and collaborative efforts for addressing such, leaders can build self-confidence and work toward improving personal and organizational performance (Albert et al., 2022).
Fostering empathy and connection	Coaches help current/emerging leaders develop empathy and build genuine connections with others by having them practice active listening, show vulnerability, and understand the role of emotional intelligence (Auerbach, 2024).
Role modeling authenticity	Through everyday interactions or coaching conversations, current/emerging leaders provide honest feedback, seek feedback, and demonstrate consistent behaviors (Culture Works HR, 2023).
Embracing risk-taking	Coaches can support current/emerging leaders to foster resilience and adapt their leadership approach to different situations in order to influence change. Porter (2018) put forth the following “homerun” statement to keep in mind when working with leaders in this area: “Taking risks involves moving forward despite fear and/or uncertainty. Until you experience discomfort, real growth and development do not exist. Realizing that failure leads to success when you learn from those mistakes will allow you to take risks more often” (para. 3).
Empowering others	Coaches can help current/emerging leaders develop coaching skills to foster stronger communication. They can also help the leader develop strategies for their team members, encourage effective delegation, and encourage team learning opportunities (Lancefield, 2023).
Measuring impact (see Table 6.2)	Coaches can help current/emerging leaders assess the impact of their leadership behaviors on team performance, employee engagement, and organizational outcomes by integrating assessment and evaluation methods.

(Continued)

Focus Area	Application
Developing others	Coaching encourages current/emerging leaders to invest in the development of their team members, both professionally and personally—preparing the next generation of leaders. By providing feedback, mentorship, and opportunities for growth, leaders can empower others to reach their full potential and contribute to organizational success (Bashir, 2023).
Development of adaptive skills	Coaching provides current/emerging leaders with the opportunity to develop adaptive skills. This may include communication skills, emotional intelligence, active listening, and conflict resolution skills, all of which are critical for effectively responding to the needs of team members in different situations.

Note: This is not an all-encompassing list, but rather a guide.

Leadership Assessments

Assessment and evaluation are two necessary elements of effective leadership. Chapter two presented several assessments focusing on leadership big picture elements. This section presents assessments specific to the aforementioned leadership behaviors. It's essential to choose an assessment that aligns with your client's or organization's specific needs and objectives (Table 6.2). Interpret the results in conjunction with other sources of information, such as feedback from colleagues, direct reports and supervisors, as well as observed behaviors. Additionally, the creation and evaluation of a development plan is required in order for change to take place.

TABLE 6.2 Leadership Assessment Tools

Assessment	Overview
Authentic Leadership Questionnaire (ALQ)	Measures four components of authentic leadership: (a) self-awareness, (b) transparency, (c) balanced processing, and (d) internalized ethical/moral perspective (Avolio et al., 2024). This valid, reliable tool contains 16 items measured on a 5-point frequency Likert scale.
Multifactor Leadership Questionnaire (MLQ)	The MLQ, developed by Bass and Avolio, is a 45-item assessment that measures a variety of leadership styles on a 6-point frequency Likert scale, but identifies the identifies the traits and characteristics of transformational leadership (2024)
MLQ + ALQ	As the name implies, this instrument merges the MLQ and ALQ. It is a 61-item assessment measuring frequency of behaviors on a 6-point Likert scale (Bass et al., 2024).

(Continued)

TABLE 6.2 Leadership Assessment Tools (*Continued*)

Assessment	Overview
Leadership Practices Inventory (LPI)	This assessment measures frequency of exemplary leadership behaviors based on the five practices of exemplary leadership. It is a 30-item assessment that utilizes a 10-point Likert scale (The Leadership Challenge, 2024).
Leadership Circle Profile (LCP)	Hailed as one of the most comprehensive 360 leadership assessments on the market, the LCP measures creative competencies and reactive tendencies (Leadership Circle, 2025). This assessment does require a certified practitioner or third party to administer.

Summary

Transformational, authentic, and situational leadership are indispensable in nursing as they promote empowerment, trust, adaptability, and ethical conduct, ultimately enhancing the well-being of the workplace. Importantly, and as mentioned above, the title of leader is not reserved for those who hold a formal administrative title; leaders are threaded throughout every layer of an organization, and each individual leadership behaviors/practices have the potential to influence the organization at large (Bass & Avolio, 1994). Thus, both the leader–coach and the individual staff or team member must understand that their leadership behaviors can have far-reaching impact. Development in such behaviors can yield an array of positive benefits.

Resources

Discussion/Reflection Questions: Coaching + Leadership

- What experiential learning opportunities can the coach utilize to assist the client who wishes to build their situational leadership competencies?
- How does coaching facilitate self-reflection and increase a leader's awareness of their strengths, weaknesses, and blind spots?
- What type of coaching would be most effective in helping current/emerging leaders gain deeper insights into their leadership behaviors and practices?
- Why is it important for the nurse leader to coach the nonformal leader on leadership behaviors and practices?

References

Abane, J. A., Adamtey, R., & Ayim, V. O. (2022). Does organizational culture influence employee productivity at the local level? A test of Denison's culture model in Ghana's local government sector. *Future Business Journal*, 8(1), 34. https://doi.org/10.1186/s43093-022-001455

Alessa, S. G. (2021). The dimensions of transformational leadership and its organizational effects in public universities in Saudi Arabia: A systematic review. *Frontiers in Psychology, 12*, https://doi.org/10.3389/fpsyg.2021.682092

Albert, N. M., Pappas, S., Porter-O'Grady, T., & Malloch, K. (2022). *Quantum leadership: Creating sustainable value in health care* (6th ed.). Jones and Bartlett.

AlMazrouei, H. (2023, February 23). Authentic leadership: Supporting employees' performance, creativity, involvement in decision-making and outcomes. *IntechOpen*. doi: 10.5772/intechopen.108624

Auerbach, J. (2024, March 29). *How to coach for empathetic leaders*. College of Executive Coaching. https://www.executivecoachcollege.com/research-and-publications/how-to-coach-for-empathetic-leadership.php

Avolio, B. J., Gardner, W. L., & Walumbwa, F. O. (2024). *Authentic leadership questionnaire*. Mind Garden. https://www.mindgarden.com/69-authentic-leadership-questionnaire#horizontalTab2

Baquero A. (2023). Authentic leadership, employee work engagement, trust in the leader, and workplace well-being: A moderated mediation model. *Psychology Research and Behavior Management, 16*, 1403–1424. https://doi.org/10.2147/PRBM.S407672

Bashir, M. (2023, May 30). *Mentoring and coaching: Building the next generation of leaders*. Forbes Coaches Council. https://www.forbes.com/sites/forbescoachescouncil/2023/05/30/mentoring-and-coaching-building-the-next-generation-of-leaders/?sh=33ed714728e9

Bass, B. M. (1990). From transactional to transformational leadership: Learning to share the vision. *Organizational Dynamics, 18*(3), 19–31. https://doi.org/10.1016/0090-2616(90)90061-S

Bass, B. M., & Avolio, B. J. (1994). Transformational leadership and organizational culture. *International Journal of Public Administration, 17*(3–4), 541–554. https://doi.org/10.1080/01900699408524907

Bass, B. M. & Avolio, B. J. (2024). *Multifactor leadership questionnaire*. Mind Garden. https://www.mindgarden.com/16-multifactor-leadership-questionnaire

Bass, B. M., Avolio, B. J., Gardner, W. L., & Walumbwa, F. O. (2024). *Multifactor leadership questionnaire + authentic leadership questionnaire*. Mind Garden. https://www.mindgarden.com/185-multifactor-leadership-questionnaire-authentic-leadership-questionnaire#horizontalTab2

Brigden, B. (2022, October 14). Situational leadership: What it is, benefits, and more. Teamwork.com. https://www.teamwork.com/blog/situational-leadership/

Broome, M., & Marshall, E. (2021). *Transformational leadership in nursing* (3rd ed.). Springer Publishing.

Cande, S. (2022, March 7). *Why being valued at work matters*. LinkedIn. https://www.linkedin.com/pulse/why-being-valued-work-matters-sam-cande#:~:text=Feeling%20valued%20at%20work%20is,relationship%20between%20employer%20and%20employee

The Center for Leadership Studies. (2024). *The right leadership, at the right time*. https://situational.com/situational-leadership/

Culture Works HR. (2023, December 21). *Role models in leadership: Why they're important and how to be one*. LinkedIn. https://www.linkedin.com/pulse/role-models-leadership-why-theyre-important-how-one-c2ytc

Deeb, I. (2023). Is training what made and nurtured transformational leaders? *Open Journal of Leadership, 12*, 324–351. https://doi.org/10.4236/ojl.2023.123016https://www.scirp.org/journal/paperinformation?paperid=127902

Duarte, A. P., Ribeiro, N., Semedo, A. S., & Gomes, D. R. (2021). Authentic leadership and improved individual performance: Affective commitment and individual creativity's sequential mediation. *Frontiers in Psychology, 12*, 675749. https://doi.org/10.3389/fpsyg.2021.675749

Harris, J.L., Roussel, L.A., & Thomas, P. L. (2022). *Clinical nurse leaders beyond the microsystem: A practical guide*. Jones & Bartlett.

Iskamto, D. (2023). Organizational culture and its impact on employee performance. *International Journal of Management and Digital Business, 2*(1). https://doi.org/10.54099/ijmdb.v2i1.584

Khan, H., Rehmat, M., & Butt, T. H. (2020). Impact of transformational leadership on work performance, burnout and social loafing: A mediation model. *Future of Business, 6*(40). https://doi.org/10.1186/s43093-020-00043-8

Kleynhans, D. J., Heyns, M. M., & Stander, M. W. (2022). Authentic leadership and flourishing: Do trust in the organization and organizational support matter during times of uncertainty? *Frontiers in Psychology, 13*, doi: 10.3389/fpsyg.2022.955300

Kouzes, J. M., & Posner, B. Z. (2017). *The leadership challenge* (6th ed.). John Wiley & Sons.

Ladika, S. (2021, July 30). *How a lack of trust undermines employee engagement*. Society for Human Resource Management. https://www.shrm.org/topics-tools/news/all-things-work/trust-never-important

Leadership Circle. (2025). *Leadership circle profile*. https://leadershipcircle.com/leadership-assessment-tools/leadership-circle-profile/

Lancefield, D. (2023, March 20). 5 strategies to empower employees to make decisions. *Harvard Business Review*. https://hbr.org/2023/03/5-strategies-to-empower-employees-to-make-decisions

Lowe, T. (2021). *The 4 keys to authentic leadership*. LinkedIn. https://www.linkedin.com/pulse/4-keys-authentic-leadership-dr-taunya-a-lowe/

Melnyk. M., & Raderstorf, T. (2021). *Evidence-based leadership, innovation, and entrepreneurship in nursing and healthcare*. Springer Publishing.

Melnyk, B. M., & Fineout-Overholt, E. (2019). *Evidence-based practice in nursing & healthcare: A guide to best practice* (4th ed.). Wolters Kluwer

Menguin, J. (2024, January 15). *The power of authentic leadership*. Strategic Learning. https://www.strategiclearning.asia/authentic-leadership/#:~:text=Authentic%20leaders%20set%20the%20tone,but%20a%20way%20of%20being.

Mind Tools Content Team. (2024a). *Transformational leadership*. https://www.mindtools.com/alj9lad/transformational-leadership

Mind Tools Content Team. (2024b). *Coaching to explore beliefs and motives*. https://www.mindtools.com/awvx8r7/coaching-to-explore-beliefs-and-motives

Pasaribu, S. B., Goestjahjanti, F. S., Srinita, S., Novitasari, D., & Haryanto, B. (2022). The role of situational leadership on job satisfaction, organizational citizenship behavior (OCB), and employee performance. *Frontiers in Psychology. 13*, doi: 10.3389/fpsyg.2022.896539

Peters, B. (n.d.). *Three steps to strengthen your self-awareness.* The Coaching Lab. https://www.theleadershipcoachinglab.com/blog/steps-to-strengthen-your-self-awareness

Porter, H. (2018, January 11). *You win or you learn: Risk taking for leaders.* Forbes Coaches Council. https://www.forbes.com/sites/forbescoachescouncil/2018/01/11/you-win-or-you-learn-risk-taking-for-leaders/?sh=602c9aeb3e5c

Quality Improvement Center for Workforce Development. (2022). *Transformational leadership.* https://www.qic-wd.org/umbrella-summary/transformational-leadership

https://ijbssnet.com/journals/Vol_8_No_2_February_2017/19.pdf

Riggio, R. E. (2014, January 22). What is authentic leadership? Do you have it? *Psychology Today.* https://www.psychologytoday.com/us/blog/cutting-edge-leadership/201401/what-is-authentic-leadership-do-you-have-it

Rogers, K. (2018). *Do your employees feel respected?* Harvard Business Review. Do Your Employees Feel Respected?

Shick, M. (2023). *Authenticity: How authentic leadership reshapes organizational culture in project management.* International Institute for Learning [Blog]. https://blog.iil.com/authenticity-how-authentic-leadership-reshapes-organizational-culture-in-project-management/

Steinmann, B., Klug Hannah, J. P., & Maier Günter, W. (2018). The path is the goal: How transformational leaders enhance followers' job attitudes and proactive behavior. *Frontiers in Psychology, 9*, https://www.frontiersin.org/articles/10.3389/fpsyg.2018.02338

Wolf, J. (2022, July 15). *Situational leadership: What it is and how to build it.* BetterUp. https://www.betterup.com/blog/situational-leadership-examples#:~:text=Situational%20Leadership%C2%AE%20means%20adapting,Leadership%C2%AE%20Theory%20in%201969

Ystaas, L. M. K., Nikitara, M., Ghobrial, S., Latzourakis, E., Polychronis, G., & Constantinou, C. S. (2023). The Impact of Transformational Leadership in the Nursing Work Environment and Patients' Outcomes: A Systematic Review. *Nursing Reports (Pavia, Italy)*, *13*(3), 1271–1290. https://doi.org/10.3390/nursrep13030108

CHAPTER 7

COACHING TO BUILD STRONGER TEAMS

This chapter will discuss team coaching. Content will include discussion on what constitutes a high-performing team and the link among team performance, professional, and organizational outcomes.

Chapter Objectives

1. Review the foundations of teamwork
2. Explore high-performing teamwork
3. Articulate how to apply coaching principles and practices to build strong, high-performing teams

Teamwork

Teamwork, broadly speaking, refers to a collaborative effort put forth by members of any group or department within an organization to achieve a common goal. Teams must be able to work cooperatively, contribute ideas, assume/share responsibilities, welcome diverse opinions, customs, or preferences, and actively participate in group decision-making efforts. In any team, collaboration is essential for meeting the teams' goals and objectives, but within the healthcare workforce, interprofessional collaborative practice is equally, if not more so, critical for workplace success (Department of Labor, n.d.).

Interprofessional collaboration begins with interprofessional education. The Interprofessional Education Collaborative (IPEC), first established in 2009, currently consists of 22 national health organizations across the healthcare disciplines—including the NLN and AACN (IPEC, 2023). Their work, as the name implies, encompasses interprofessional education and collaborative practice. This is IPEC's statement on interprofessional education and practice:

> Interprofessional education occurs when students from two or more professions learn about, from, and with each other to enable effective collaboration and improve health outcomes. Once students understand how to work in an interprofessional

> capacity, they are ready to enter the workplace as a member of the collaborative practice team. This is a key step in moving health systems from fragmentation to a position of strength (IPEC, para. 1, n.d.).

IPEC has outlined the following four core competencies, along with 33 sub-competencies, for individuals in collaborative practice:

- Values and ethics
- Roles and responsibilities
- Communication
- Teams and teamwork

Incorporation of these core competencies, as well as the sub-competencies, aims to develop both student and working professionals' collaborative practice, which will in turn improve workplace satisfaction, patient satisfaction, and quality-of-care delivery. As IPEC's core goal is to introduce these competencies during healthcare training (e.g., higher education and clinical rotations and entry-level practice), both academicians and hospital leaders alike need to model and promote these collaborative practices to cement the foundation for teamwork within their respective departments. In addition, leaders need to execute effective leadership practices (e.g., transformational) and reinforce the notion that no one individual, irrespective of how exceptional, is better, stronger, or more productive than the team (Broome & Marshall, 2021). Even more so, leaders must have the ability to function as a coach because coaching influences team-based outcomes (Nyfoundi et al., 2023), which can be a determining factor in whether teams are high-performing teams.

High-Performing Teams

High performing teams are those who share common vision, values, goals, and strategies to overcome challenges and achieve superior business results (Lean Agility, 2022). A high-performing team is characterized by the same skills/behaviors as traditional teams, with added attributes that contribute to the team's effectives, productivity, innovation, creativity, and overall success. These additional attributes include leadership trust—both within the team and outside the team—moving beyond SMART goals, adaptability, conflict resolution, and incorporation the 5C's model of high-performing teams.

Leadership Trust Inside and Outside the Team

Strong leadership drives strong performing teams; it is done by shifting from a self-oriented mindset to an outward, employee-centered mindset (Chhaya, 2024; SHRM, 2024). By doing this, leaders establish trust among their staff, which leads to trust in the organization and improves engagement, productivity, and creativity (Friedman, 2024). Trust is also an essential component *within* high-performing teams. It is the foundation and is modeled after the team's external leader (e.g., chief executive). In fact, emerging literature suggests that trust is the differentiating factor between standard work teams and high-performing teams and that it contributes to shared leadership. Additionally, a recent study including over 1,000 U.S. workers, identified five additional characteristics for how high-performing teams build trust to ensure success: (a) describing *how* collaboration will take place, (b) proactively sharing information, (c) sharing credit, (d) embracing disagreement, and (e) embracing a growth mindset (Friedman, 2024).

According to Friedman's (2024) study, high-performing teams are more likely to discuss what their expertise or areas of interest is in regard to a particular project, their communication preferences, and previous experiences that may or may not have been successful in the past. They are willing to work together to identify each member's strengths and preferences, rather than assigning tasks and partnerships based on the team leader's assumptions or preconceived notions regarding member–member compatibility.

Also highlighted in the study was the notion that being proactive with information sharing and transparency fosters trust among teams and increases team performance. Proactive knowledge sharing allows team members to feel empowered and supports/promotes psychological safety, creating a culture of inclusion. Additionally, high-performing teams not only give members credit where credit is due, but they also share their recognition of a job well done with one another; after all, it is the work of the team that results in an accomplishment. Sharing credit and recognition is not only motivating, but also empowering, which are two critical pillars to team success. Although leaders may have different perspectives on what constitutes a high-performing team—including team skills, outcomes, member contributions, or adaptive capacity—actual team members may measure their performance based on effectiveness, synergy among members, or comparability to other teams within their own industry (Albert et al., 2022; Friedman, 2024).

Lastly, high-performing teams, within this particular study, "believe that workplace disagreements lead to better decisions" (Friedman, 2024, p. 5). These teams believe that conflict should be viewed as a strength, which, in turn, assists the team in taking stronger initiative in collectively solving the problem. Members of a high-performing team also proactively address tension, especially if they feel they are creating it—a differentiating factor from traditional teams.

Moving Beyond SMART Goals

High-performing teams do not excel by operating on a linear process or line; rather, they operate "on a moving matrix similar to a slide puzzle that can move up and down and side-to-side based to two primary factors: team trust and team aim" (American Public Human Services Association, 2010, p. 2). Trust within teams is a fundamental element that cannot be overstated. Trust makes members feel safe, heard, and supported, while providing an opportunity to push boundaries—for example, experiment with innovation and creativity (American Public Human Services Association, 2010).

As noted in previous chapters, goals should have clarity and specificity (Albert et al., 2022), which can be achieved by using a SMART goal framework. The level of difficulty, or ambition, of the goal is equally important to specificity, leading to greater effort toward reaching the actual goal, which, in turn, can positively impact performance (Locke & Latham, 2002; SHRM, 2024). But, ensuring every member of the team understands their individual role, path, or strategy toward achieving the goal will help solidify the aim, assist in interdependence, and further add trust between members (SHRM, 2024). So, while it is critical to establish a goal that represents the core values and customer-driven objectives of the respective organization, the aim is what connects the team together and results in action planning toward achieving the goal.

Adaptability

In today's fast-paced environment, change is constant. Whether it's market dynamics, technological advancements, or shifts in customer needs, teams must be able to pivot quickly and effectively (New Jersey Institute of Technology, 2024). This adaptability is what enables the team to not only navigate, but effectively problem-solve. Teams that are adaptable can approach problems with flexibility, encourage collaboration and creativity, inspire innovation, and build team efficacy and confidence (New Jersey Institute of Technology, 2024). Moreover, adaptability contributes to team resilience, allowing members to maintain their composure and focus, find ways to overcome difficulties, and emerge stronger and more united.

Conflict Resolution Skills

Conflict is normal in both personal and professional contexts. However, how conflict is managed separates traditional teams from high-performing teams. Furthermore, conflict resolution requires understanding different perspectives, staying calm under pressure, and focusing on finding mutually beneficial solutions, rather than assigning blame. By utilizing techniques such as de-escalation, collaboration, and clear, concise communication, individuals can turn conflicts into opportunities for growth (See Chapter 9 for more on conflict resolution).

5C's Model of High-Performing Teams

These additional attributes align and/or compliment Peter Hawkins's model, the 5C's model of high-performing teams. Hawkins, a renowned professor, author, thought leader, and cofounder of the Global Team Coaching Institute, developed five disciplines or capacities of high-performing teams. These five disciplines or capacities include (a) commission, (b) clarifying, (c) cocreating, (d) connecting, and (e) core learning.

In brief, the first *C*—commission—explores whether the team is clear about who and what stakeholders such as a board, customers, community, investors, etc. require (Hawkins, 2014). According to Hawkins (2014), commission is about understanding the *"why"* (*e.g.*, *why* we are here). Next, clarifying is evaluating the *"what."* A high-performing team evaluates their own collective skills, expertise, and experiences and reflects upon how these attributes can be brought together to create a collective endeavor—moving beyond parallel contribution (Hawkins, 2014). The third *C*, cocreating, also known as the *"how,"* is all about understanding how the team can move beyond precooked thoughts and inspire innovative, creative thinking among one another. Connecting, the fourth *C* is all about generating and spreading enthusiasm both inside and outside the team boundaries. Last, core learning concerns the learning and development needs of the entire team—not just the individuals within it; it is about collective learning, growth, and development. More information on Hawkins's model can be found here:

https://www.leadershipcentre.org.uk/artofchangemaking/theory/5-capacities-of-high-performance-teams/

Learning Checkpoint

What is the foundation of a high-performing team?

High-Performing Teams: Professional and Organizational Outcomes

High-performing teams can provide personal and professional advantages for employees who are part of the team, as well as contribute to enhanced productivity, innovation, and ultimately, organizational success. High-performing teams can influence a member's professional outcomes by highlighting and leveraging each member's strengths and skill sets to help them perform at peak capacity, potentially uncovering an unknown potential. Because high-performing teams embrace diverse perspectives and differing opinions, members who may not be used to working with inclusivity and belonging can add this new skill set to their own leadership toolbox, which is an asset required for formal and/or executive leadership roles and adds value to the current talent pipeline, establishing strategies for diversity, equity, and inclusion within the workplace (Project Management Institute, 2023; Rodriguez-Ojeda, 2023).

High-performing teams that create a culture of psychological safety can encourage members to share new ideas both inside and outside the team, increase transparency, and cultivate internal accountability by taking ownership of their tasks and responsibilities. Furthermore, psychological safety can foster honesty and vulnerability and lessen team conflict (Patil et al., 2023). In addition, the aforementioned characteristics can be transferred outside of the team to impact varying aspects of the members' respective career (Project Management Institute, 2023).

Working in a high-performing team provides a sense of accomplishment, and the collaborative and supportive nature of these teams can boost morale and empowerment. Empowerment can provide an opportunity for individual skill or behavioral development. When a member seeks to foster their own growth and development (e.g., emotional intelligence negotiation, persuasion, etc.), they promote an environment of learning, which can positively influence retention, engagement, satisfaction, and the long-term success of the organization (Tenney, 2024). Thus, high-performing teams play a crucial role in driving professional outcomes by enhancing productivity, fostering innovation, improving decision-making, and contributing to a positive organizational culture.

However, while the idea of creating or sustaining high-performing teams is attractive for leadership, leaders must be in tune to the team's collective functionality based on characteristics of high-performing teams (e.g., trust, goal clarity, etc.). If any of the aforementioned characteristics are not observed within a team, leadership intervention should follow. The intervention will depend on the need(s). In addition, intervention is needed when a leader identifies the presence of any of the following 10 barriers to high-performing teams (SHRM, 2024):

- Nonparticipating leadership
- Poor decision-making
- Infrequent/poor communication
- Diversity not valued
- Lack of mutual trust
- Inability to manage/navigate conflict
- Lack of goal clarity
- Poorly defined roles/responsibilities
- Relationship issues
- Negative atmosphere

Nurse Leaders: Application of Coaching to Build High-Performing Teams

Although some may argue that nursing is outside the realm of a traditional, high-performing team as discussed above, there are different types of high-performing teams, including parallel teams, project teams, management teams, and virtual teams (SHRM, 2024). In brief, both project and management teams are more business oriented, with project teams focusing on a new product or service, and management teams focusing on the performance of the department. Virtual team members never meet in person but collaborate via communication technology platforms to achieve an organizational initiative. Parallel teams are comprised of individuals from varying departments or units (often sharing the same background, such as nursing) to collaborate and intervene on improvement-oriented activities (e.g., evidence-based practice quality improvement (EBPQI)). Thus, nursing fits into the high-performing team category. However, members must be coachable, preferably as a team, before they can be deemed a high-performing team.

Team coaching follows the same principles and practices as traditional, individual coaching. It involves a structured yet flexible process that is tailored to the unique needs of the team and can be applied in various contexts to drive success and growth. By focusing on building trust, enhancing communication, achieving team goals, and fostering continuous improvement, coaching can help teams reach their full potential and objectives. It is a powerful tool for developing high-performing teams.

To facilitate the team coaching process, the leader–coach should select a framework they are familiar with that suits the team's needs. As a refresher from Chapter 2, we will examine *some* easy to use and popular models for the leader–coach, manager, and novice coach.

GROW

GROW is one of the more common, widely used coaching models that requires the coach to establish a clear goal, assess the reality of the current situation, encourage exploration and brainstorming on strategies or solutions for moving forward, and put those strategies or solutions into a feasible, attainable action plan (Polemis, n.d.). Polemis (n.d.) provides a list of starter questions for each element within this model to assist the coach in facilitating the coaching conversation. Though some of these questions may appear to be geared to the one-to-one coaching conversation, they can be easily applied or adapted for team coaching. To see more, view the following link:

https://wp.nyu.edu/coaching/tools/grow-model/

ACHIEVE

The ACHIEVE model, which was not presented in Chapter 2, can be considered an expansion of the GROW model of coaching, and it can be easily applied by a novice coach, leader, or manager during leadership or conversations centered on coaching. This model has seven steps, including the following:

1. Assess the current situation within the team
2. Brainstorm creatively (explore *what* needs to be changed)
3. Hone in on the goal(s) (identify goals and objectives)
4. Initiate option generation (explore *how* things can be changed)
5. Evaluate options (rank the options)
6. Plan valid actions (plan the steps and sub-steps to complete the overall plan)
7. Encourage momentum (maintain follow-up meetings and progress check-ins)

To learn more, view the following link:

https://worldofwork.io/2019/08/the-achieve-coaching-model/#:~:text=The%20ACHIEVE%C2%AE%20coaching%20model,plan%20design%20and%20Encourage%20Momentum

CLEAR

CLEAR is another commonly used, easy-to-integrate model that requires the coach to establish an agreement ensuring all members are aligned and committed to being coached. The model includes actively listening about the problem or opportunity of interest, exploring where the clients are in relation to their current state versus desired state, developing action plans (in this case, team-oriented plans), and regularly reviewing progress and outcome measures (Leadership Centre, 2024).

OSKAR

The OSKAR solution-focused model emphasizes the importance of partnership, collaboration, and celebration of achievements. This model can help individuals and teams change behavior and produce noticeable organizational change. To see more, view the following:

https://www.mindtools.com/agrk092/the-oskar-coaching-framework

Choosing the right coaching framework depends on the team's specific needs and the desired outcomes. The GROW, ACHIEVE, CLEAR, and OSKAR models offer valuable, easy-to-use frameworks for team-based coaching, and the chosen model can be adapted to fit the unique needs of the nursing team and its respective units or departments.

Importantly, teams are only as good their leaders, leaders internal and external to the team. Leaders can positively influence their team's outcomes by establishing trust, setting clear goals, fostering collaboration, providing targeted, team-based training, and encouraging continuous improvement. Leaders must also ensure that every member of the team understands their own individual role, path, or strategy toward achieving the team's goal. Finally, leaders must always strive to apply the golden rule of coaching—more listening and less talking—to help ensure that every individual and the team as a whole feel they are part of the solution.

Let's consider some example scenarios where performance coaching can be applied with the healthcare team using one of the coaching frameworks above.

Interdisciplinary Team Collaboration

Example: Improving patient care coordination

- **Scenario:** A hospital wants to enhance collaboration among its interdisciplinary teams (e.g., doctors, nurses, therapists, and social workers) to improve patient care coordination.
- **Coaching application:**
  - **Assessment:** Conduct initial assessments through surveys and interviews to understand the current state of collaboration and identify specific challenges.
  - **Goal setting:** Meet with the team to review data findings and set specific goals, such as improving the timeliness of patient discharges.
  - **Facilitation and training:** Organize regular team meetings facilitated by an external coach or the nurse leader serving as the coach to discuss patient cases, share information, and develop coordinated action-oriented plans to meet the set goal(s). Provide training sessions or professional development opportunities to facilitate the growth and development of the team. Sessions should be focused on open-ended questioning to inspire intellectual stimulation and empowerment, with *most* of the discussion being generated from the team.
  - **Feedback and reflection:** Implement a system for continuous feedback and reflection after each patient discharge to learn what worked well and what needs improvement.

Nursing Team Development

Example: Enhancing nursing staff morale

- **Scenario:** A hospital nursing unit is experiencing low morale and high turnover rates.
- **Coaching application:**
  - **Assessment:** Conduct surveys and focus groups to identify the main issues affecting morale and turnover.
  - **Brainstorming/innovation sessions:** Meet with the nursing team to collectively discuss what can be done to mitigate the situation. The team should take the lead, and the coach should ask thought-provoking questions to maintain the team's momentum in the brainstorming/innovation sessions.
  - **Goal setting:** Establish goals such as improving job satisfaction and reducing turnover rates.
  - **Begin to generate a team-based action plan:** Explore how to bridge the gap between the current state and the desired state. At this stage, all options should be deemed viable and recorded (e.g., professional development, mentorship programs, enhanced clinical ladder program, incivility training, wellness rooms, greater flexibility with scheduling, etc.).
  - **Rank options:** Rank the list of options generated from the team-based action plan from most favored, feasible, applicable, to the least.
  - **Operationalize the action plan:** Determine how and when to operationalize the plan.
  - **Team-building activities and regular check-ins:** Organize team-building activities to strengthen relationships and foster a supportive work environment. Regular check-ins with the coach or leader–coach should also be scheduled to discuss progress, address concerns, adjust strategies as needed, and encourage momentum.

Patient-Centered Care Teams

Example: Implementing patient-centered care practices

- **Scenario:** A healthcare organization wants to shift to a more patient-centered care model.
- **Coaching application:**
  - **Contracting:** Unite the team with the focus of the problem of interest or opportunity.
  - **Assessment:** Conduct patient and staff surveys to understand current perceptions and practices related to patient-centered care.

- **Goal setting:** Set goals to improve patient satisfaction scores and enhance patient engagement.
- **Action planning:** Offer training workshops focused on patient-centered communication, empathy, and shared decision-making to familiarize the team with the new practice model. Collaborate with the team to develop systems to integrate patient feedback into care planning and improvement initiatives into the current workflow.
- **Team collaboration:** Facilitate regular interdisciplinary team meetings.
- **Evaluation and adjustment:** Continuously evaluate the effectiveness of patient-centered care initiatives and adjust strategies based on feedback and outcomes.

Summary

Coaching to build stronger teams requires leaders to recognize their impact on team performance and outcomes. It also requires a strong sense of trust. Trust is the foundation for collaboration, communication, conflict resolution, accountability, and flexibility. It is the glue that holds the team together and what differentiates a traditional work team from a high-performing team. Coaching to build stronger teams involves the same fundamental principles as traditional coaching—assessment, goal setting, evaluation, and follow-up—but differs slightly with focus, approach, and outcomes measurement being based on the collective performance of the team.

Resources

Case Examples

Read the following scenarios and draft a response on how a teams-based approach can solve the problem. Please include principles and coaching frameworks discussed in this chapter to develop your coaching approach to solving the problem.

1. **Elevating Curriculum Development**
    - Scenario: A nursing faculty team is tasked with overhauling the nursing curriculum to better prepare students for the complexities of modern healthcare systems.
    - Approach:
    - Evaluation: How will you know if your approach was effective? What are your outcomes? How will you measure them?

2. **Improving Student Retention and Success**
    - Scenario: The nursing program is experiencing challenges with student retention and success rates, particularly among underrepresented groups.
    - Approach:
    - Evaluation: How will you know if your approach was effective? What are your outcomes? How will you measure them?
3. **Creating High-Performing Student Project Teams**
    - Scenario: In a graduate program, students are required to complete a capstone project in teams, but some teams struggle with collaboration and meeting project deadlines.
    - Approach:
    - Evaluation: How will you know if your approach was effective? What are your outcomes? How will you measure them?
4. **Enhancing Diversity, Equity, and Inclusion (DEI) Initiatives**
    - Scenario: A university aims to strengthen its DEI efforts across campus, particularly within academic departments and student organizations.
    - Approach:
    - Evaluation: How will you know if your approach was effective? What are your outcomes? How will you measure them?
5. **Administrative Leadership Teams**
    - Scenario: The leadership team of a university's administrative department is tasked with improving the institution's student services.
    - Approach:
    - Evaluation: How will you know if your approach was effective? What are your outcomes? How will you measure them?

Coaching scenarios were generated using Chat GPT.

References

American Public Human Services Association. (2010). *Building high performing teams*. University of Wisconsin-Madison. https://media.wcwpds.wisc.edu/website-docs/wcwpds/org-development/oe/2-Building-High-Performing-Teams-Trust-Aim-full.doc

Albert, N. M., Pappas, S., Porter-O'Grady, T., & Malloch, K. (2022). *Quantum leadership: Creating sustainable value in health care* (6th ed.). Jones and Bartlett.

Broome, M., & Marshall, E. (2021). *Transformational leadership in nursing* (3rd ed.). Springer Publishing.

Chhaya, N. (2024, April 8). 5 well intentioned behaviors that can hurt your team. *Harvard Business Review*. https://hbr.org/2024/04/5-well-intentioned-behaviors-that-can-hurt-your-team

Department of Labor. (n.d.). *Teamwork*. teamwork.pdf (dol.gov)

Friedman, R. (2024). How high performing teams build trust. *Harvard Business Review.* https://hbr.org/2024/01/how-high-performing-teams-build-trust

Hawkins, P. (2014, November 3). *The 5 disciplines of high performing teams.* Kogan page. https://www.koganpage.com/hr-learning-development/the-5-disciplines-of-high-performing-teams

Interprofessional Education Collaborative (IPEC). (n.d.). *What is interprofessional education?* (as cited in World Health Organization, 2010, *Framework for action on interprofessional education & collaborative practice*). https://www.ipecollaborative.org/about-us

Interprofessional Education Collaborative (IPEC). (2023, November 20). *IPEC core competencies for interprofessional collaborative practice: Version 3.* https://www.ipecollaborative.org/assets/core-competencies/IPEC_Core_Competencies_Version_3_2023.pdf

Leadership Centre. (2024). *Transformational coaching.* https://www.leadershipcentre.org.uk/artofchangemaking/theory/transformational-coaching-the-clear-model/

Lean Agility. (2022). *High performing teams.* https://leanagility.com/en/high-performing-teams

Locke, E. A., & Latham, G. P. (2002). Building a practically useful theory of goal setting and task motivation: A 35-year odyssey. *American Psychologist, 57*(9), 705–717. https://doi.org/10.1037/0003-066X.57.9.705

New Jersey Institute of Technology. (2024, March 16). *Six reasons why high-performance teams should learn how to adapt and change* [Blog]. https://continuedlearning.njit.edu/six-reasons-why-high-performance-teams-should-learn-how-adapt-and-change

Nyfoundi, M., Shipton, H., Theodorakopoulos, N., & Budhwar, P. (2023). Managerial coaching skill and team performance: How does the relationship work and under what conditions? *Human Resource Management Journal, 33*(2), 328–345. DOI: 10.1111/1748-8583.12443

Patil, R., Raheja, D., Nair, L., Deshpande, A., & Mittal, A. (2023). The power of psychological safety: Investigating its impact on team learning, team efficacy, and team productivity. *The Open Journal of Psychology, 16,* DOI: 10.2174/18743501-v16-230727-2023-36

Polemis, J. (n.d.). *The GROW framework.* Coaching for Leadership. The GROW Framework – Coaching for Leadership

Project Management Institute. (2023, November). *Building and leading high-performing teams.* https://www.pmi.org/learning/thought-leadership/building-high-performing-teams

Rodriguez-Ojeda. (2023, August 25). Creating a culture of DEI starts with leadership. Forbes Financial Council. *Forbes.* https://www.forbes.com/sites/forbesfinancecouncil/2023/08/25/creating-a-culture-of-dei-starts-with-leadership/

Society for Human Resource Management (SHRM). (2024). *Developing and sustaining high performing teams.* https://www.shrm.org/topics-tools/tools/toolkits/developing-sustaining-high-performance-work-teams

Tenney, M. (2024). *Why a learning culture is so important for success* [Blog]. PeopleThriver. https://businessleadershiptoday.com/why-is-a-learning-culture-important/

CHAPTER 8

COACHING TO BUILD EMPLOYEE DEVELOPMENT (PART I)

This chapter will discuss one critical area of employee development: communication. Nurse leaders will learn valuable tools and techniques that can be applied in the workplace to foster employee development in the area of communication. However, before leaders can develop their employees' communication skills, they must first understand their own strengths, weaknesses, and approaches to mastering communication.

Chapter Objectives

1. Examine one's communication practices
2. Analyze the importance of emotional intelligence in communication practices
3. Apply coaching to foster simple, strong communication

Communication

Communication, arguably one of the most important leadership skills, can be loosely defined as an exchange of information between individuals (Merriam-Webster, n.d.). The National Communication Association adds to this by asserting that "Communication focuses on how people use *messages* to generate meanings within and across various contexts ..." (NCA, 2024, para. 1). So, leaders should strive for effective delivery. Effective communication is crucial in many areas, including personal relationships, workplaces, education, healthcare, and public affairs. It promotes networking and relationship building across all these areas; it is an absolute essential element for every leader.

As we all know, communication can occur in various forms, including verbal, nonverbal, and digital (emails, texts, social media). Effective communication involves not just the transmission of a message but also ensuring that the message is understood by the receiver as intended by the sender, which requires clear, concise delivery. For current and emerging leaders, mastery of the fundamentals of communication, including quantity or calibration of communication, can greatly influence how others view their leadership abilities (Broome & Marshall, 2021). Flynn and Lide (2023) found that leaders are 10 times as likely to be criticized for undercommunicating. Additionally, leaders who are viewed as undercommunicating are more likely to be perceived as ill-qualified for their leadership role (Flynn & Lide, 2023).

With this understanding, it is important to take a moment to examine one's communication style/abilities to see where improvement is needed. Box 8.1 demonstrates a short communication self-assessment.

Box 8.1: Communication Self-Assessment

Instructions: Reflect on your communication practices, and rate yourself on a scale of 1 to 5:
1 = Strongly Disagree, 2 = Disagree, 3 = Neutral, 4 = Agree, and 5 = Strongly Agree
Reflect on your ratings to note areas for improvement.

1. **Clarity of message**
   a. **I clearly articulate my ideas and instructions.**
   Rating: ___
   Reflection: ________________________________
   b. **I avoid using jargon or overly complex language when communicating with my team.**
   Rating: ___
   Reflection: ________________________________
   c. **I organize my thoughts logically before speaking.**
   Rating: ___
   Reflection: ________________________________
2. **Active listening**
   a. **I demonstrate active listening by paraphrasing or summarizing what others say.**
   Rating: ___
   Reflection: ________________________________
   b. **I ask clarifying questions to ensure I fully understand others.**
   Rating: ___
   Reflection: ________________________________
   c. **I provide feedback that shows I have understood the concerns or suggestions of others.**
   Rating: ___
   Reflection: ________________________________
   d. **I give advice and direction when I should be allowing others an opportunity to generate ideas.**
   Rating: ___
   Reflection: __________________________

3. **Tone and delivery**
   a. **I use an appropriate tone of voice for different situations.**
      Rating: ___
      Reflection: ______________________________
   b. **I maintain an engaging and motivating presence when speaking to my team.**
      Rating: ___
      Reflection: ______________________________
   c. **I vary my pitch and volume to maintain interest and emphasize key points.**
      Rating: ___
      Reflection: ______________________________
4. **Nonverbal communication**
   a. **My body language (e.g., gestures, posture) supports/mirrors the message I am delivering.**
      Rating: ___
      Reflection: ______________________________
   b. **I make appropriate eye contact when communicating.**
      Rating: ___
      Reflection: ______________________________
   c. **My body language (e.g., leaning in, head nodding) supports/demonstrates that I am engaged in the conversation.**
      Rating: ___
      Reflection: ______________________________
5. **Adaptability and responsiveness**
   a. **I adapt my communication style to fit my audience (e.g., adjusting language or tone based on the listener's level of understanding).**
      Rating: ___
      Reflection: ______________________________
   b. **I remain calm and composed when faced with communication barriers or misunderstandings.**
      Rating: ___
      Reflection: ______________________________
6. **Persuasion and influence**
   a. **I effectively persuade and influence others through clear and compelling communication.**
      Rating: ___
      Reflection: ______________________________
   b. **I provide strong, evidence-based arguments to support my points.**
      Rating: ___
      Reflection: ______________________________

7. **Emotional intelligence in communication**
   a. **I consider the emotional state of others when communicating important information.**
   Rating: ___
   Reflection: ____
   b. **I effectively manage my own emotions during conversations, particularly in difficult situations.**
   Rating: ___
   Reflection: ____
   c. **I acknowledge and address the emotional reactions of others during communication.**
   Rating: ___
   Reflection: ____
8. **Feedback and continuous improvement**
   a. **I regularly seek feedback on my communication skills.**
   Rating: ___
   Reflection: ____
   b. **I am open to and act on feedback to improve my communication effectiveness.**
   Rating: ___
   Reflection: ____
   c. **I reflect on my communication after key interactions and identify areas for improvement.**
   Rating: ___
   Reflection: ____

Generated using Chat GPT.

While all of the elements included in the self-assessment are crucial for effective communication, two areas weigh more heavily than others: active listening and emotional intelligence.

Active Listening

Mastery of active listening is considered to be one of the most valuable tools a leader can possess (Broome & Marshall, 2021). Additionally, active listening is a key strategy for leaders who wish to adopt a more coaching-centered style of leadership. Cuncic (2024) lists the following seven techniques to help leaders master this communication skill:

1. Being fully present in the conversation
2. Showing interest by practicing good eye contact
3. Noticing (and using) nonverbal cues (e.g., head nodding, good body posture)

4. Asking open-ended questions to encourage further responses
5. Paraphrasing and reflecting back what has been said
6. Listening to understand rather than to respond
7. Withholding judgment and advice

Importantly, leaders must demonstrate genuine interest and authenticity when implementing techniques 4 through 7. Otherwise, leaders risk being perceived as inauthentic (Broome & Marshall, 2021), which can yield negative results.

Emotional Intelligence

There are different models of emotional intelligence, and this text discussed Genos model of emotional intelligence in early chapters. However, Daniel Goleman's current model of emotional intelligence (redesigned in the early 2000s) cannot go without mention, especially in regard to communication. Goleman's model is perhaps one of the most widely recognized models, breaking emotional intelligence into four domains: (a) self-awareness, (b) self-management, (c) social awareness, and (d) relationship management. The model is further divided into 12 competencies, which are not defined in this text (Goleman, 2011). Because emotional intelligence is embedded into every word, action, decision, and behavior of our everyday lives, it is important to understand the definition and role that each component plays in leadership. Goleman's domains are presented in Table 8.1.

TABLE 8.1 Goleman's Model of Emotional Intelligence

Component	Definition	Role in Leadership
Self-Awareness	The ability to recognize and understand your own emotions, needs, drives, and strengths, and weaknesses (Goleman, 2011; Ott, n.d.).	Self-awareness allows leaders to understand how their emotions impact their thoughts, behavior, and interactions with others.
Self-Management	The ability to control, redirect, or channel emotions and impulses in useful ways to create a safe and trusting environment (Goleman, 2011; Ott, n.d.).	Leaders who manage their emotions effectively can maintain calm and clarity in stressful situations, enabling them to think and act constructively. Self-management also involves being adaptable and resilient, qualities that help leaders navigate challenges and inspire confidence in others.

(Continued)

TABLE 8.1 **Goleman's Model of Emotional Intelligence (*Continued*)**

Component	Definition	Role in Leadership
Social Awareness	The ability to understand the emotions, needs, and concerns of others; the ability to read and respond to emotional cues (Ott, n.d.) and be cognizant of the potential impact of the environments—external (surrounding) and internal (feelings of others at a given time).	Recognizing social and organizational dynamics enables leaders to navigate complex situations effectively.
Relationship Management	The ability to develop and maintain good relationships and successfully manage social interactions by incorporating the other three components (Ott, n.d.).	Leaders who excel in this area are skilled at building strong, cooperative relationships, managing conflicts constructively, and driving collective success.

Generated using Chat GPT.

Emotional intelligence is integral to effective communication, particularly in leadership. Emotional intelligence ensures that the messaging is clear, easily understood, takes into account the emotional state of the audience, and enhances the leader's awareness of the external climate (e.g., the surrounding environment to ensure conditions are appropriate for conversation or coaching). Leaders with high emotional intelligence are better equipped to communicate, manage, inspire, coach, and develop their teams. Therefore, an emotional intelligence self-assessment is warranted. Though there are a variety of emotional intelligence self-assessments on the market, many deeply elaborate and providing a wealth of information, they do come at a cost. However, we can take a basic look at the fundamentals in Box 8.2, which is similar to the communication self-assessment in Box 8.1.

Box 8.2: Emotional Intelligence Self-Assessment

Instructions: Reflect on your leadership practices, and rate yourself on a scale of 1 to 5:
1 = Strongly Disagree, 2 = Disagree, 3 = Neutral, 4 = Agree, and 5 = Strongly Agree
Reflect on your ratings to note areas for improvement.

1. **Self-awareness**
   a. **I am aware of my emotions and how they affect my thoughts and behavior.**
      Rating: ___
      Reflection: ________________________________

   b. **I understand my strengths and weaknesses and use this knowledge to guide my actions.**
      Rating: ___
      Reflection: ______________________________
   c. **I am confident in my abilities and have a strong sense of self-worth.**
      Rating: ___
      Reflection: ______________________________
2. **Self-management**
   a. **I remain calm and composed even in stressful situations.**
      Rating: ___
      Reflection: ______________________________
   b. **I manage my emotions and impulses effectively, avoiding rash decisions or actions.**
      Rating: ___
      Reflection: ______________________________
   c. **I am comfortable with ambiguity and change.**
      Rating: ___
      Reflection: ______________________________
   d. **I take initiative and am proactive in pursuing opportunities and meeting goals.**
      Rating: ___
      Reflection: ______________________________
   e. **I have the ability to mobilize my own emotions.**
      Rating: ___
      Reflection: ______________________________
3. **Social awareness**
   a. **I can easily identify the feelings of others.**
      Rating: ___
      Reflection: ______________________________
   b. **I am aware of the social and political dynamics within my organization and navigate them effectively.**
      Rating: ___
      Reflection: ______________________________
   c. **I prioritize understanding and meeting the needs of my team and other stakeholders.**
      Rating: ___
      Reflection: ______________________________
   d. **I build bonds with colleagues and network whenever possible.**
      Rating: ___
      Reflection: ______________________________
4. **Relationship management**
   a. **I communicate clearly and effectively, ensuring that my messages are understood by others.**
      Rating: ___
      Reflection: ______________________________

b. **I am skilled at resolving conflicts in a way that is constructive and maintains positive relationships.**
   Rating: ___
   Reflection: ______________________________
c. **I coach others to help them reach goals.**
   Rating: ___
   Reflection: ______________________________
d. **I work well in teams, fostering collaboration and helping to build a strong team dynamic.**
   Rating: ___
   Reflection: ______________________________

Generated using Chat GPT.

Learning Checkpoint

After completing the emotional intelligence assessment, what was most surprising? What was least surprising?

Approaches to Improve Communication

Though there are a myriad of resources that offer tips, tricks, and strategies for enhancing communication, the Center for Creative Leadership (2024) put forth 15 basic, easy-to-apply principles to help leaders enhance or master their communication skills. They include the following:

1. Communicate relentlessly
2. Set the tone—be crystal clear with expectations
3. Be simple and direct
4. Use stories to illustrate the message
5. Always be prepared
6. Know the audience
7. Don't rely on words alone—use body language with intent
8. Read the room
9. Use powerful questions to learn what the audience is thinking and feeling
10. Encourage input
11. Seek feedback on the message
12. Affirm with actions
13. Initiate the tough or challenging conversations
14. Involve others before developing plans of action
15. Remember your reputation

To read more about each of these, visit the following link:

https://www.ccl.org/articles/leading-effectively-articles/communication-1-idea-3-facts-5-tips/

Written communication is as equally important as spoken communication. Therefore, it is important to note that digital etiquette is one element missing from the Center for Creative Leadership's list. Though leaders can—and absolutely should—leverage technology in their communications with staff, they must remember and utilize the *basic principles* (that many seem to forget) to ensure they are maintaining professionalism and maximizing the message. These principles include the following:

- Avoid sending internal messages through text messaging
- Be mindful that digital communication lacks nonverbal cues (be thoughtful as to how your message will be perceived)
- Use emojis sparingly in email or video conferencing platforms (to avoid misinterpretation of boundaries)
- Respect response times (especially when working within different time zones)
- Acknowledge receipt (if you can't respond immediately, acknowledge receipt and indicate when you'll follow up)
- Choose the right medium (use email for formal communication, secure messaging apps for quick queries, and video calls for detailed or collaborative discussions)
- Use professional presentation in video calls:
    - Dress appropriately (virtual meetings are still professional meetings)
    - Ensure a clean background
    - Mute when not speaking
- Encrypt confidential information (use encryption tools for sharing sensitive documents)
- Use a secure network
- Be cautious with links and attachments (avoid clicking on suspicious links or downloading unexpected attachments)
- Respect status indicators (e.g., "Do not disturb")
- Be aware of cultural differences (understand that digital communication norms may vary across cultures)
- Be mindful of digital fatigue

By optimizing digital etiquette, leaders and team members can enhance communication, reduce misunderstandings, and foster a more positive and productive work environment.

How to Apply Coaching to Foster Simple, Strong Communication

Once leaders have mastered their communication skills, they can begin to develop the needed skills in their staff. Leaders who invest in developing their staff's communication skills not only improve individual performance but also foster a more collaborative and productive work environment. A coaching approach is particularly effective in this regard, as it enables personalized development, continuous improvement, and the creation of a culture that encourages open communication.

Identify the Problem or Opportunity of Interest

The first step in using a coaching approach to enhance communication skills is to identify the specific needs of each staff member. This can be achieved through self-assessments, peer feedback, and one-on-one discussions. Understanding each individual's strengths and areas for improvement allows leaders to tailor coaching strategies to meet those needs. This personalized approach ensures that coaching efforts are focused and relevant, leading to more significant improvements.

Establish Goals

Once communication needs are identified, leaders should work with staff to set clear, achievable goals. These goals should be created using a goal framework (e.g., SMART). For example, a "general" goal might be to improve active listening skills or to demonstrate leadership boundaries in written communication (this could be for a charge nurse, coordinator, etc.). The leader should further probe the staff member to add a measurement and time frame. Using the first example, the goal could be refined. One example would be to use reflection and paraphrasing (one piece of active listening) during the next three meetings specifically, followed by seeking feedback from colleagues to ensure this was observed. To demonstrate leadership boundaries in written communication, the goal could be to specifically reduce the number of emojis and exclamations in team updates by 30% before the next month. By setting clear goals with measurable outcomes, leaders can help staff achieve their overarching goals (Leonard & Watts, 2024).

Tailor Coaching Plans

A coaching approach to leadership requires leaders to establish individualized coaching plans (not to be confused with remediation plans) that focus on the specific communication skills each staff member needs to develop. These plans should include practical exercises, such as role-playing scenarios, reflective listening drills, and opportunities for staff to practice these skills in real work situations. Leaders should ask probing questions about progress to prompt critical thinking and self-reflection. They should also provide feedback when necessary. Though the feedback loop is crucial for continuous development, the leader should ensure that the feedback is a two-way process (Hirsch, 2020)—with the staff speaking more than the leader.

It is key for coaches to ensure that a safe and supportive environment has been established. This, in turn, will ease anxiety and enhance staff comfort. Leaders should also instill a judgment-free zone, as judgment can inhibit progress. Also, it is a must to celebrate small wins (Laker, 2024). Leaders should acknowledge progress and improvements to bolster confidence and encourage ongoing practice/execution. However, as with any skill development or behavior change, ongoing opportunities for learning, such as additional training courses or access to digital tools may be required and recommended as needed. Regular check-ins should be scheduled to allow leaders an opportunity to monitor progress, goal status, and to make adjustments.

Consider Group Coaching and Peer Feedback

In addition to one-on-one coaching, group coaching sessions can be highly effective in building communication skills. Workshops focused on specific aspects of communication, such as public speaking or conflict resolution, provide a collaborative environment for learning. Encouraging peer feedback within these sessions also fosters a culture of open communication and continuous learning. These can take place in the settings of "lunch and learns" or they can be integrated into professional development blocked time.

Model and Encourage Reflective Practice

As with other skills, it is essential for leaders to model effective communication. By demonstrating clear, concise, and respectful communication in all interactions and mediums, leaders set the standard for their teams. Additionally, leaders should encourage reflective practice for staff to regularly evaluate their communication experiences. This can be facilitated through journaling or post-meeting reflections.

Summary

Communication is one of the most important leadership skills to master. While a multitude of elements are crucial for effective communication (see self-assessment Box 8.1), active listening and emotional intelligence are front and center. Thus, without a firm understanding of one's baseline communication skills, leaders cannot effectively articulate their vision, set clear expectations, or inspire and motivate their teams.

Resources

Discussion/Reflection Questions

1. How do you typically approach giving feedback to a colleague or direct report? How could you adjust your approach to encompass more of a coaching element?
2. What strategies can you use to become a more active listener?
3. What role does emotional intelligence play in effective communication?
4. What role does emotional intelligence play in coaching?
5. How can the nurse leader build their team's communication skills using a coaching approach?

References

Broome, M., & Marshall, E. (2021). *Transformational leadership in nursing* (3rd ed.). Springer Publishing.

Center for Creative Leadership. (2024, August 26). *Essential communication skills for leaders*. https://www.ccl.org/articles/leading-effectively-articles/communication-1-idea-3-facts-5-tips/

Cuncic, A. (2024, February 12). *7 active listening techniques for better communication*. Very Well Mind. https://www.verywellmind.com/what-is-active-listening-3024343

Goleman, D. (2011). *Leadership: The power of emotional intelligence*. Key Step Media.

Hirsch, J. (2020, June 1). Good feedback is a two-way conversation. *Harvard Business Review*. Good Feedback Is a Two-Way Conversation (hbr.org)

Flynn, F. J., & Lide, C. R. (2023). Communication miscalibration: The price leaders pay for not sharing. *Academy of Management, 66*(4). https://doi.org/10.5465/amj.2021.0245

Laker, B. (2024, February 19). Small victories, big impact: Mastering the art of celebrating quick wins. *Forbes*. https://www.forbes.com/sites/benjaminlaker/2024/02/19/small-victories-big-impact-mastering-the-art-of-celebrating-quick-wins/

Leonard, K., & Watts, R. (2024, July 9). The ultimate guide to S.M.A.R.T. Goals. *Forbes*. https://www.forbes.com/advisor/business/smart-goals/

National Communication Association. (2024). What is communication? https://www.natcom.org/about-nca/what-communication/

Ott, C. (n.d.). *What is emotional intelligence?* Ohio State University Extension. https://ohio4h.org/sites/ohio4h/files/imce/Emotional%20Intelligence%20Background.pdf

Merriam-Webster. (n.d.). *Merriam-Webster.com dictionary*.

CHAPTER 9

COACHING TO BUILD EMPLOYEE DEVELOPMENT (PART II)

This chapter will focus on conflict resolution. Conflict cannot and should not be avoided; rather, it should be viewed as an opportunity for growth and development. When managed properly, conflict can improve relationships and aid in individual self-development. Thus, in this chapter, nurse leaders will learn valuable tools and techniques that can be applied to fostering employee development.

Chapter Objectives

1. Examine types of conflict
2. Examine types of conflict resolution
3. Articulate how to address conflict through coaching

Types of Conflict

Albert et al. (2022) published a thought-provoking "point to ponder" in their book *Quantum Leadership: Creating Sustainable Value in Healthcare.* The text states:

> About 90% of the average leader's responsibilities involve dealing with human behavior and human interaction. Given that this is true, why do leaders spend so little time learning how to resolve issues that arise out of human dynamics? (Albert et al., 2022, p. 221).

Could this be because leaders don't truly understand the types of conflict? Do they think conflict is mostly self-resolvable? Or is it because conflict management isn't their "area of expertise" so they avoid learning about it? While there are many reasons that leaders spend little time learning how to resolve issues, leaders must understand that their conflict resolution strategies are detrimental to the success of their unit or department and can seep into the organization at large. Although this text does not aim to make nurse leaders experts at conflict identification or resolution, it does present fundamental elements that are required for successful leadership. Although there are varying types of conflict—anywhere between three and seven, depending on the source—this text, will review three types of conflict, including (a) interpersonal, (b) intra-personal, and (c) task. This brief review will set the stage for understanding how/when to apply, teach, or coach others on conflict resolution strategies.

Interpersonal Conflict

Interpersonal conflict refers to a conflict that occurs between two or more individuals due to a multitude of factors. *Some* of these factors include lack of communication, inappropriate communication style, power differentials (e.g., asserting dominance), lack of support, passive-aggressive behaviors, ethical disputes, role conflict, and incivility (Albert et al., 2022; ANA, 2023; Angelo, 2019). Interpersonal conflict should be addressed as it arises; letting it fester can yield a negative impact on the team.

Intrapersonal Conflict

This type of conflict occurs *within* an individual, impacting one's mental peace (Elmoudden, 2023). It occurs when one struggles with dilemmas or competing desires. Sources for this type of conflict can include misperceptions of other's beliefs or values, race, culture, political views, and low PsyCap (Albert et al., 2022). Addressing and managing intrapersonal conflict can yield a positive impact on decision-making, mental health, and overall well-being (Elmoudden, 2023).

Task Conflict

Task conflict arises when there is an issue or disagreement over workplace tasks. Such tasks include things like work assignments, deadlines, inconsistent application of policy or procedure, or resource allocation (Shonk, 2024a). Task conflict can be beneficial if managed well. It can stimulate critical thinking, innovation, and collaboration.

Understanding the different types of conflict are fundamental in identifying the root issues, applying the appropriate resolution strategies, and utilizing coaching strategies to establish creative solutions to neutralize or capitalize on the conflict (ANA, 2023).

Types of Conflict Resolution

Researchers Kenneth Thomas and Ralph Kilmann studied, observed, and ultimately pioneered one of the most widely recognized conflict management models—the Thomas Kilmann conflict resolution model. This model, which ultimately became a conflict assessment known as the TKI (Thomas-Kilmann

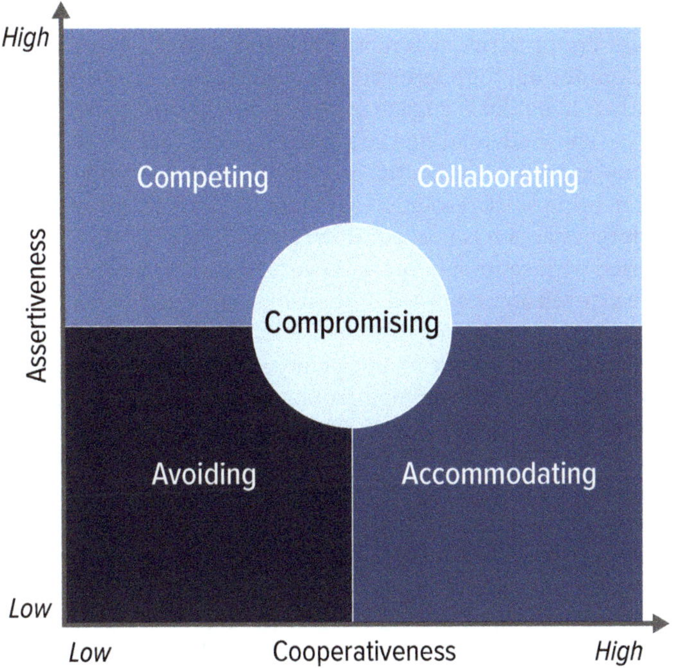

FIGURE 9.1 Thomas-Kilmann Conflict Model

Instrument) encompassed five core conflict handling modes, or styles (McPheat, 2022). This model assesses one's response to conflict based on their five core conflict handling modes and the degree to which they cooperate and/or demonstrate assertiveness (Figure 9.1).

The Five Modes

Each conflict resolution mode has its advantages and disadvantages. Consider the following five modes of conflict resolution:

1. **Avoiding, low assertiveness, and low compromising** occurs when individuals avoid conflict in its entirety (McPheat, 2022). Although this mode has its time and place (e.g., when the issue is trivial or when emotions are too high for productive discussion) it also leaves unchecked, unresolved issues, tasks, and/or emotions. This, in turn, provides an opportunity for resentment to build, contributing to an unhealthy work culture.
2. **Accommodating, low assertiveness, and higher compromising** leads one to "cave," "take the L",or agree to disagree and accept the other person's opinion or stance on the topic at hand (McPheat,

2022). Individuals may opt for this mode if the conflict is minor or preserving harmony is more important than the issue.

3. **Competing, high assertiveness, and low compromising** occurs when individuals engage in debate, and/or assume an argumentative stance defending their point of view (McPheat, 2022). It's a power-driven mode, often used in high-stakes situations. This mode can bring quick resolution to urgent or emergent situations or when decisive action is needed. However, this style of relating should be used with caution because if overused or misused, competing can lead to tension, damaged relationships or reputations, and may foster a win–lose mentality (McPheat, 2022).
4. **Compromising**, the middle point, occurs when an individual works diligently to find common ground or a mutually agreed upon solution (Myers-Briggs, 2024). Thus, in this mode, neither party gets everything they want, but both get something. It is an efficient mode for conflict resolution that preserves relationships and leads to a moderate level of satisfaction for both parties. However, one must be cautious not to utilize this mode exclusively; sometimes other modes, like collaborating, can yield more benefits (McPheat, 2022).
5. **Collaborating, highly assertive, and highly cooperative** requires both parties to work together to collectively solve the issue. Collaboration encourages open communication, builds stronger relationships, and inspires creativity and innovation (McPheat, 2022). Although this is a valuable conflict resolution mode, it can be time-consuming and resource intensive and requires a high level of trust (McPheat, 2022).

Applying Conflict Management Skills

Conflict should not be avoided or suppressed; rather, it should be viewed as a means for growth and transformation (Albert et al., 2022). Using conflict management skills such as communication, constructive persuasion and negotiation, and appreciative leadership, can help teams achieve maximum performance.

Communication

Communication in such teams requires the focus to be on *coaching*, allowing for open, candid conversations (SHRM, 2024). These types of conversations promote openness and trust, and ultimately, less unnecessary conflict (see Chapter 8 for more on communication).

Constructive Persuasion and Negotiation

Constructive persuasion is not a sales pitch per se, but it's a process of negotiating a shared solution (Conger, 1998). According to Conger (1998), there are four essential steps to effective constructive persuasion, including

(a) credibility, (b) persuasive framing, (c) providing evidence, and (d) emotional connection.

Credibility is a result of trust among team members, which can be fostered by establishing/building relationships and by sharing or demonstrating expertise in the industry. Expertise is a critical factor for constructive persuasion because buy-in for product, service, policy/procedure change will be necessary. There are always differing viewpoints within teams, but how these viewpoints are acknowledged and navigated makes the difference in the cohesion of the team. Team members self-reflect on where their strengths/weaknesses align in regard to industry expertise and collegial relationships to enhance the outcomes and performance of the team as a whole (Conger, 1998).

Persuasive framing is the second element of effective constructive persuasion, and it can be achieved by identifying and highlighting shared beliefs or advantages amongst the team members. This is a fundamental skill of a transformative leader, and each member of the team can capitalize on this skill when collaborating on team projects (Conger, 1998). In some circumstances, there may not be an easily identifiable or even a shared belief within reach. It is important for one to recognize when it is time to go back to the drawing board to redefine project goals and outcomes and collaborate to adjust the team's position to meet the needs of the department or system.

Next is building the case with evidence. Though healthcare is a champion of evidence-based practice and evidence-based decision-making, teams presenting evidence to stakeholders, or even other members, should make their case compelling. To do this, the team should use convincing language with imagery, stories, and analogies to support their numerical data. This adds an edge and can be fruitful in optimizing the effectiveness of the presentation and driving change (Conger, 1998).

The last step is emotional connection. Emotions, whether intentional or not, come into play in the decision-making process. According to Oehler (n.d.) decisions carry emotions because decisions come with some degree of risk. Decision making should be forward facing (e.g., about the future) and the future can be uncertain. This uncertainty adds an additional emotional element to the decision-making process.

Each member of the team must acknowledge their emotional connection to the decision-making process and align these emotions with their target audience (Conger, 1998). Thus, to be an effective, constructive persuader, individuals (or teams) must have a deep sense of how their colleagues within the department or system will react to the proposition being put forth.

In addition to constructive persuasion is the need for negotiation skills. As healthcare continues to be in a perpetual state of limited resources, clinicians, managers/leaders, teams, and executives need to have a set of fundamental tools (negotiation skills) to maximize or reallocate resources to meet department or system needs (Clay-Williams et al., 2018). Miller (2023) highlights six negation skills that are critical for any professional in any industry, including

(a) communication (which was presented above), (b), emotional intelligence, (c) planning, (d) value creation, (e) strategy, and (f) reflection.

According to Miller (2023) and the above depiction, communication requires active listening, civil discussion and the ability to clearly and succinctly articulate the argument—either for or against the proposition at hand. Emotional intelligence, which is threaded throughout every aspect of one's personal and professional life, requires one to be in tune with their own emotions and how these emotions impact interactions and decision-making. Understanding others' ideas, position, or perception is a critical component to this aspect of leadership, whether leading outside a team or leading from within a team.

Planning ahead is critical to any negotiation. Miller (2023) asserts that the first component of the planning should be establishing the bargaining zone, also known as the zone of possible agreement (ZOPA), which can be positive or negative. A positive bargaining zone is a zone with overlapping consensus. A negative zone occurs when there is no overlapping consensus. Trying to get an advantage occurs in the negative bargaining zone. In business this is called the best alternative to a negotiated agreement (BATNA). BATNA, as first described by Fisher et al. (1991) in *Getting to Yes: Negotiating Agreement Without Giving In*, keeps one (or a team) from leaving the table empty-handed. Here is an example of a BATNA that is provided by the American Academy of Family Physicians (AAFP) and authored by Swedlund (2023, p. 12):

> Dr. Taylor is a third-year resident considering career options. She is interested in teaching medical students and publishing on medical education. She already has an offer from a community health system for a full-time clinical role at a guaranteed salary of $235,000. She is currently talking to a recruiter for a local academic health system about another position with 80% clinical care, 10% teaching time, and 10% time to support academic output, which offers a guaranteed salary of $220,000. The academic job is more ideal for her, but knowing that she has the BATNA of the full-time clinical job to fall back on, Dr. Taylor pushes the academic health system hard in salary negotiations and they agree to increase her guaranteed salary to $240,000.

This professional role negotiation example is often used when describing a BATNA because it can be broadly applied. When establishing or using a BATNA, Shonk (2024b) describes a few important items to consider, including the following:

1. Don't reveal a weak BATNA
2. Don't bluff about your BATNA
3. Don't reveal your BATNA too early
4. DO work actively to improve your BATNA
5. Don't let anyone talk you out of your BATNA

The AAFP provides an easy to read, broad toolkit for negotiating that can be applied/transferred to the nursing discipline. To read more, view the following article:

https://www.aafp.org/pubs/fpm/issues/2023/0500/physician-negotiation.pdf

Making the best of your negotiation and ensuring the other party leaves with something is known as value creation. Though this can be achieved when employing the BATNA, it is important to foster a collaborative future-forward relationship with those you negotiated with; it can be fruitful in the production of a relationship that can yield long-term benefits (Gavin, 2019).

Strategy is about understanding what works and what does not. This can be achieved by understanding one's role and value in the negotiation process, understanding the counterpart's vantage point(s), and establishing a self-check in. This will ensure that one is staying the course within the negotiation process (Miller, 2023). Lastly, like all good leadership skills, competencies, or initiatives, engagement in self-reflection after the process is vital to fostering negotiation skills, particularly with a BATNA.

Appreciative Leadership

Appreciative leadership targets optimistic possibility (Ganguly & RoyBardhan, 2020). This leadership focuses on identifying and building upon the strengths, positive attributes, and potential of individuals, teams, and organizations. Rather than concentrating on problems or deficiencies, appreciative leaders promote positive performance and believe employees have the internal resources needed to execute tasks efficiently and effectively (Ganguly & RoyBardhan, 2020; Malloch & Porter-O'Grady, 2022). Appreciative leadership encompasses five key elements or strategies, including (a) inquiry, (b) illumination, (c) inspiration, (d) integrity, and (e) inclusion (Corporation for Positive Change, 2024; Ganguly & RoyBardhan, 2020).

1. **Inquiry:** Appreciative leaders ask questions that focus on strengths, successes, and possibilities. By doing so, they foster a culture of curiosity, learning, and positive thinking. This, in turn, creates an environment where individuals and teams participate in future facing thinking (Roussel et al., 2023, p. 119).
2. **Illumination:** Illumination is the process in which leaders help individuals recognize and determine the best ways to make a contribution (Baptise, 2017). In other words, leaders help people recognize and amplify their strengths and unique contributions so that they can achieve personal and professional goals.

3. **Inspiration:** These leaders motivate and inspire people by articulating a compelling vision of the future. They emphasize shared purpose and values, helping individuals and teams see the larger meaning in their work. They provide a sense of direction that yields hope and "unleashes energy" (Corporation for Positive Change, 2024).
4. **Integrity:** Appreciative leaders act with authenticity, transparency, and respect. They align their actions with their values, fostering trust and encouraging others to do the same (Corporation for Positive Change, 2024).
5. **Inclusion:** Appreciative leaders create inclusive environments where diverse perspectives are valued. They actively seek input and collaboration from team members, fostering a sense of belonging, co-creation, and ownership (Corporation for Positive Change, 2024).

In essence, appreciative leadership is about creating a positive environment that unlocks the potential of both individuals and teams, guiding them toward a future filled with shared purpose and success.

Learning Checkpoint

What is known as the ZOPA? Why is this important for nurse leaders to know?

Addressing Conflict Through Coaching

Conflict is an inevitable aspect of human interactions (Albert et al., 2022). However, when managed correctly, it can lead to growth, innovation, and stronger relationships. While the previous sections of this chapter reviewed conflict type and accompanying conflict resolution strategies, this section will discuss the value of applying a coaching approach to managing/resolving conflict. As noted in the previous eight chapters of this text, coaching is a powerful development tool that can be integrated into everyday leadership practices.

Coaching for conflict resolution first involves assurance that the individual is willing to resolve the conflict. This can be done by asking the individual open-ended questions (e.g., Are you willing to put the work in to solve this conflict? How adaptable and flexible can you be during the process?). These questions will help the leader–coach gauge the participant's commitment to resolution of the conflict. Once the leader determines the individual is willing to work, they can move forward.

Next, the leader should begin to explore the individual's understanding of the conflict and their level of self-awareness. Helping individuals understand their own roles in the conflict, their triggers, and their emotional responses will be pivotal for establishing an action plan. The leader can uncover this information by engaging in further questioning. The following questions are not an exhaustive list, but they provide some possible questions:

1. What is the conflict about?
2. What is your role in this conflict? (if not answered above)
3. How did this conflict arise?
4. How do you feel about this conflict/situation?
5. Why is resolving this conflict important to you?
6. How do you envision a compromise to this conflict?
7. What requests can you ask of the other person to assist in the compromise?

It is important to keep in mind that conflict management styles between two individuals may be very different. Be sure to assess the individual's perception of how the other individual involved in the conflict behaves or presents themselves. Perception is a key element in helping to find common ground and drafting a strategy for the resolution.

Additional points of consideration for the coach (going back to the basics) include the following:

- Establishing a safe and open environment
    - Create a neutral and nonjudgmental space where both parties feel safe to express their thoughts and emotions openly. By doing so, individuals are more likely to engage in productive dialogue rather than remaining defensive or feeling hopeless.
- Focusing on interests, not positions
    - Guide individuals to focus on underlying interests and future objectives (why they want what they want). This approach helps uncover real motivations and drives creative solutions.
- Building emotional intelligence
    - Help develop emotional intelligence by increasing self-awareness, self-regulation, empathy, and social skills. This enables individuals to manage their emotions better and understand the emotions of others, which is crucial for resolving conflicts.
- Developing conflict resolution skills
    - Give opportunity for individuals to learn and practice conflict resolution techniques such as those covered in this chapter. This empowers them to handle future conflicts more effectively.
- Creating accountability and action plans
    - Help individuals develop action plans for resolving conflicts. Help individuals identify specific steps they can take to address the issues and hold them accountable for following through. Conflict assessments may be utilized as well; however, some of these assessments have a cost (e.g., TKI).

Summary

Conflict resolution is a fundamental skill of leadership. It requires leaders to understand basic conflict types, root causes of a conflict, and conflict resolution styles/approaches. Leaders can utilize conflict resolution skills, such as communication, constructive persuasion and negotiation, and appreciative leadership to mitigate unwanted conflict, build stronger relationships, and enhance team dynamics.

Resources

Case Example 1: Conflict in a Clinical Setting

In a hospital setting, a nurse leader observed ongoing tension between two nurses over work assignments. Tamika felt that Matthew was avoiding difficult tasks, while Matthew felt that Tamika was being overly critical and controlling. The nurse leader, acting as a coach, scheduled one-on-one coaching sessions with each nurse. During these sessions, the leader encouraged self-reflection and helped both nurses identify their own roles in the conflict. Tamika realized that her critical nature was partly driven by her perfectionism, while Matthew acknowledged that he was avoiding difficult tasks because of a lack of confidence.

Then, in a joint coaching session, the nurse leader facilitated a conversation in which both nurses practiced active listening, expressed their concerns, and clarified their needs. The leader guided them to focus on shared goals rather than their individual frustrations. Together, they developed a plan for distributing tasks more equitably and agreed on ways to support each other as they moved forward.

- List three to five questions the nurse leader could have asked to help both nurses identify their own roles in the conflict.

    1.
    2.
    3.
    4.
    5.

- List three to five questions the nurse leader could have asked to help both nurses identify a shared goal.

    1.
    2.
    3.
    4.
    5.

- What would the next step be for the nurse leader in ensuring this conflict was resolved?

Case Example 2: Conflict in an Academic Setting

In an academic department, Associate Professor Dr. Patel and Department Chair Dr. Tenzen had a disagreement about workload allocation. Dr. Patel believed that her teaching assignments were being "shuffled" compared to others in the department, who had a more consistent teaching schedule, and subsequently felt she was being "pushed out".

An external coach was brought in to work with both parties (this was not the first time Dr. Tenzen has had conflicts with his team). In individual coaching sessions, the coach encouraged both Dr. Patel and Dr. Tanzen to reflect on their goals, assumptions, and emotions. Dr. Patel came to understand that her feelings of frustration were linked to her perception of being undervalued, while Dr. Tanzen recognized that his approach to teaching assignment distribution might not have been communicated clearly enough. However, after a few more meetings, the coach realized that each professor's approach to resolving the conflict was vastly different.

- List three to five questions the coach could have asked to help Dr. Patel come to the realization that she felt undervalued.

  1.
  2.
  3.
  4.
  5.

- List three to five questions the coach could have asked to help Dr. Tanzen determine his communication was ineffective.

  1.
  2.
  3.
  4.
  5.

- Knowing that the two individuals have a vastly different conflict resolution approach, how might the coach proceed with resolving this conflict?

- What would the action plan look like for this scenario?

Coaching scenarios were generated using Chat GPT.

Discussion/Reflection Questions

- What is constructive persuasion?
- What is a BATNA?
- Think of a time you had to engage in a negotiation. Did you present your BATNA? If not, why not?
- Appreciative leadership encompasses five elements/strategies. Please list one way that you as the leader–coach could demonstrate each of these elements/strategies.
- Describe a time when you utilized a coaching approach to solve a conflict.
- What type of coaching approach would be best to apply when working with conflict? Explain your answer.

References

Albert, N., Pappas, S., Porter-O'Grady, T., & Malloch, K. (2022). *Quantum leadership: Creating sustainable value in health care* (6th ed.). Jones & Bartlett Learning.

American Nurses Association (ANA). (2023, September 18). *Conflict resolution strategies for nurse leaders.* https://www.nursingworld.org/content-hub/resources/nursing-leadership/conflict-resolution-in-nursing/#:~:text=Nursing%20conflict%20resolution%20requires%20patience,that%20provides%20quality%20patient%20care.

Angelo, E. (2019). Managing interpersonal conflict: Steps for success. *Nursing Management, 50*(6), 22–28. https://doi.org/10.1097/01.NUMA.0000558479.54449.ed

Baptise, M. (2017). *Appreciative leadership: 5 core strategies.* LinkedIn.

Clay-Williams, R., Johnson, A., Lane, P., Li, Z., Camilleri, L., Winata, T., & Klug, M. (2018). Collaboration in a competitive healthcare system: negotiation 101 for clinicians. *Journal of Health Organization and Management, 32*(2), 263–278. https://doi.org/10.1108/JHOM-12-2017-0333

Conger, J. (1998, May–June). The necessary art of persuasion. *Harvard Business Review.* https://hbr.org/1998/05/the-necessary-art-of-persuasion#:~:text=Effective%20persuasion%20involves%20four%20distinct,vivid%20language%20and%20compelling%20evidence.

Corporation for Positive Change. (2024). *Five strategies of appreciative leadership.*

Elmoudden, S. (2023). Teaching intrapersonal conflict: A necessity in a post COVID world. *International Journal on Social and Education Sciences, 5*(3), 736–745. https://doi.org/10.46328/ijonses.583

Fisher, R., Ury, W. L., & Patton, B. (1991). *Getting to yes: Negotiating agreement without giving in*. Penguin Books.

Ganguly, M., & RoyBardhan, M. (2020). *Role of appreciative leadership in organizational development: The roadmap to employee growth*. IGI Global Scientific Publishing. DOI: 10.4018/978-1-5225-9675-2.ch013

Gavin, M. (2019, March 5). *3 ways to create value in negotiation*. Harvard Business School Online. https://online.hbs.edu/blog/post/negotiation-tactics-how-to-add-value

Goleman, D. (2011). *Leadership: The power of emotional intelligence*. Key Step Media.

Malloch, K., & Porter-O'Grady, T. (2022). *Appreciative leadership: Building sustainable partnerships for healthcare*. Jones & Bartlett Learning.

McPheat, S. (2022, October 4). *What is the Thomas-Kilmann conflict management model?* Management Training Specialists (mtdtraining.com).

Miller, K. (2023, May 11). *6 negotiation skills all professionals can benefit from*. Harvard Business School Online. https://online.hbs.edu/blog/post/negotiation-skills

The Myers-Briggs Company. (2024). *Managing conflict to drive positive change*. Thomas-Kilmann Conflict Mode Instrument (TKI®).

Oehler, K-H. (n.d.). *What do emotions have to do with decision making?* Dension. https://denisonconsulting.com/transform/article-emotions-decision-making/

Roussel, L., Thomas, P. L., & Harris, J. L. (2023). *Management and leadership for nurse administrators* (9th ed.). Jones & Bartlett.

Shonk, K. (2024a, August 29). *3 types of conflict and how to address them*. Program on Negotiation. Harvard Law School. https://www.pon.harvard.edu/daily/conflict-resolution/types-conflict/#:~:text=Different%20types%20of%20conflict%20%E2%80%94%20including,different%20approaches%20to%20conflict%20resolution.&text=In%20the%20workplace%2C%20it%20sometimes,conflict%20are%20always%20with%20us.

Shonk, K. (2024b, May 9). *BATNA examples—and what you can learn from them*. Program on Negotiation.

Society for Human Resource Management (SHRM). (2024). *Developing and sustaining high performing teams*. https://www.shrm.org/topics-tools/tools/toolkits/developing-sustaining-high-performance-work-teams

Swedlund, M. (2023). *Negotiation for physicians: Practical strategies to improve Bargaining Success*. American Academy of Family Physicians. https://www.aafp.org/pubs/fpm/issues/2023/0500/physician-negotiation.pdf

CHAPTER 10

RESOURCES FOR COACHING

This chapter provides leaders with resources, tools, and activities that will help facilitate the application of coaching within the workplace.

Coaching Programs

As noted in earlier chapters, the ICF is an internationally recognized organization for coaches and coaching. In addition to the abundance of resources for novice and seasoned coaches, those looking to obtain certification for career advancement or those interested in becoming internal or external coaches can take the step of participating in an accredited ICF coaching program. To explore accredited programs, leaders can utilize the education search service feature within the ICF website. The link to conduct a search is here:

The Gold Standard in Coaching | ICF - Find Education

Books

There are many great coaching books on the market. Some are focused on the conception of coaching, some are a blend of history and application, others offer tips, strategies, and share coaching experiences. As a new coach, or someone who is interested in learning more about coaching, building their coaching skills, and gaining basic resources that can be utilized in the clinical or academic settings, a few books would be of value (Table 10.1). Importantly, coaching programs often provide a list of recommended readings and resources unique to their program offerings.

TABLE 10.1 **Book List**

Title	Link
The HeART of Laser-Focused Coaching: A Revolutionary Approach to Masterful Coaching by Marion Franklin	More can be found at: https://www.amazon.com/s?k=The+HeART+of+Laser-Focused+Coaching%3A+A+Revolutionary+Approach+to+Masterful+Coaching&crid=1Y16MPO1T9ZV2&sprefix=the+heart+of+laser-focused+coaching+a+revolutionary+approach+to+masterful+coaching%2Caps%2C167&ref=nb_sb_noss
Trillion Dollar Coach: The Leadership Playbook of Silicon Valley's Bill Campbell by Eric Schmidt, Jonathan Rosenberg, and Alan Eagle	More can be found at: https://www.amazon.com/Trillion-Dollar-Coach-Leadership-Playbook/dp/0062839268
Coaching Skills: The Definitive Guide to Being a Coach by Jenny Rogers	More can be found at: https://www.amazon.com/COACHING-SKILLS-DEFINITIVE-Humanities-Counselling/dp/0335261922/ref=sr_1_1?crid=1A5L3O57ZRTEW&dib=eyJ2IjoiMSJ9.cgqh-ceKVaBu1FrVvwpnXr4t5ZP2ZI24P6FinyoJLW5cPrf7DAZRqPXLLyLVi6Vy.HJugNnwHfpsr9GHAsxwlUdOD5_UTjn1MVKFkosc6Vj8&dib_tag=se&keywords=Coaching+Skills%3A+The+Definitive+Guide+to+Being+a+Coach&qid=1726155099&sprefix=coaching+skills+the+definitive+guide+to+being+a+coach+%2Caps%2C103&sr=8-1

Title	Link
The Advice Trap: Be Humble, Stay Curious & Change the Way You Lead Forever by Michael Bungay Stanier *The Coaching Habit: Say Less, Ask More & Change the Way You Lead Forever by Michael Bungay Stanier*	More can be found at: https://www.amazon.com/Advice-Trap-Humble-Curious-Forever/dp/1989025757/ref=sr_1_1?crid=15D1BSJMX8Y2U&dib=eyJ2IjoiMSJ9.JEIlxzLQnixxPBiXU0To6gPuO-EXAoEzTI_4caWEGD_Ocj9Du0D2FKB7rZhenUC4ToY6Q4d9DEd4mI3sWqC3Xw.TiSgpsDmt7ajDq_RGoBFrnMNoLG8MwLzC0uAK3ddDcM&dib_tag=se&keywords=The+Advice+Trap+and+The+Coaching+Habit&qid=1726155131&sprefix=the+advice+trap+and+the+coaching+habit+%2Caps%2C123&sr=8-1
The Coach's Way: The Art and Practice of Powerful Coaching in Any Field by Eric Maisel	More can be found at: https://www.amazon.com/Coachs-Way-Practice-Powerful-Coaching/dp/160868864X/ref=sr_1_1?crid=3BNPMKV74AXTC&dib=eyJ2IjoiMSJ9.1PAp9JOkDs6eGeimkyqzW5LdCzDJZqY1Gd4Ctw9Guew.h9NeS4sBtk1G6sKtMObpfAhTsWH21E0i_GGjWeU0fiY&dib_tag=se&keywords=The+Coach%27s+Way%3A+The+Art+and+Practice+of+Powerful+Coaching+in+Any+Field&qid=1726155178&sprefix=the+coach%27s+way+the+art+and+practice+of+powerful+coaching+in+any+field+%2Caps%2C116&sr=8-1

Note. This is a suggested list of readings—not an exhaustive list.

Templates

For those in a leadership role, one-to-one check-ins and/or budgeted time with team members is critical in fostering the growth and development of individual members (it also plays a role in fostering the skills of the leader–coach). If the leader–coach meets with their team member in a more formal capacity, note-taking is essential. Below are a *few* essential example templates that can be utilized to help track progress.

Client/Staff Profile Sheet (Internal Coaching; Leader/Manager as Coach)

Name: ______________________________
Email: ______________________________
Work Days: ______________________________
Position: ______________________________

Opportunity of interest or problem/issue(s) to be discussed:

Why is this opportunity or problem/issue an important topic to you?

What do you wish to achieve (e.g., big-picture ending).

How will you know you've reached your outcome?

Internal Coaching Contract Template

Internal Coaching Contract

Date: ______________________________
Employee/Coachee Name: ______________________________
Department/Team: ______________________________

1. **Purpose of Coaching**
   The purpose of this internal coaching engagement is to support the coachee in ______________________________ (e.g., service excellence, networking circle, power and influence, etc.). Coaching will focus on the areas of ______________________________(e.g., self-awareness, emotional intelligence, communication, conflict resolution, etc.).

2. **Coaching Objectives**
   The specific objectives for this coaching engagement include:

   - ______________________________
   - ______________________________
   - ______________________________

   (Coachee and Coach will collaborate on defining these objectives in the first session.)

3. **Coaching Process (including Progress Evaluation)**
   - Duration and frequency: Coaching sessions will take place [weekly/biweekly/monthly] and will last approximately [30/45/60] minutes.
   - Length of coaching engagement: The coaching relationship will last for [3/6/12] months from the date of this contract.
   - Coaching medium: Sessions will be conducted in person/over phone/video conferencing (choose as appropriate).

4. **Roles and Responsibilities**
   - Coach's role: The coach will ask insightful, thought-provoking questions that will assist the coachee toward identifying solutions and strategies. The coach will not provide direct solutions or advice, but rather empower the coachee to develop their own ideas. However, if development opportunities are needed, the coach can/will provide recommendations.
   - Coachee's role: The coachee is responsible for identifying goals, being open to feedback, and implementing agreed-upon actions. The coachee agrees to fully participate, complete any homework or self-reflection exercises, and communicate openly with the coach.

5. **Confidentiality**
   The coaching relationship is confidential. The coach agrees not to disclose any information discussed during coaching sessions to anyone outside the coaching relationship without the coachee's consent, except in cases where disclosure is required by law or organizational policy (e.g., safety concerns, harassment).

6. **Accountability and Commitments**
   - The coach commits to being punctual, prepared, and engaged in all coaching sessions.
   - The coachee commits to attending all coaching sessions on time and completing any agreed-upon actions between sessions.

Signatures
Coach Signature: ______________________________
Date: ______________________________
Coachee Signature: ______________________________
Date: ______________________________

*By signing this contract, both parties confirm that they have read and understood the content within this agreement and will abide by the terms and responsibilities outlined.

Notes:
The internal coaching template may or may not be necessary, depending on the nature of the coaching (e.g., formal documentation required or useful in promotion or advancement).

This contract is a non-legal binding template that can be adjusted based on the specific requirements of the organization and the nature of the internal coaching being conducted.

Coaching Plan Template

<table>
<tr><th colspan="2">Session</th><th>Actions</th><th>Development Activities</th></tr>
<tr><td></td><td></td><td></td><td></td></tr>
<tr><td></td><td></td><td></td><td></td></tr>
<tr><td></td><td></td><td></td><td></td></tr>
<tr><td></td><td></td><td></td><td></td></tr>
<tr><td></td><td></td><td></td><td></td></tr>
</table>

Action Planning (To Be Completed by Client)

Overall goal/outcome (e.g., big-picture ending):

Short-term goal (e.g., by the end of the month I will ...):

Action Steps	Timeline	Successful completion (Y or N). If not successful, why?

Progress Tracker (Based on Action Planning Document)

Name:
Date:
Overall goal/outcome (e.g., big-picture ending):

Short-term goal (e.g., by the end of the month I will ...)

Action step (including timeline for completion)	Status	Issues encountered	Adjustment required (Y or N)	Next step	Next check-in

Topic-Based Questions

Coaching Conversations/Micro-coaching:

- What's on your mind?
- What is the real challenge here for you?
- Share with me the ideas you have to solve this challenge.
- What matters most to you in your practice?
- What talents do you know you have but are not using?
- How can you do more of the work you love?
- What actions do you need to take but are avoiding?
- What is the best way for you to receive feedback?

General/Opening Questions in a One-to-One:

- What would you like to discuss during our session today?
- What do you want to achieve?

- What makes this an important topic?
- How will you know you achieved your goal?
- What is the benefit of taking action?
- What strengths can you utilize to make this change happen?
- What are your options moving forward?
- What is the first step you can take?

Career:

- What is your dream job?
- What do you love about what you do now?
- What don't you love about what you are doing now?
- What is important to you?
- What are you passionate about?
- What are your strengths?
- What do you want in terms of your career?
- What don't you want in terms of your career?
- What are your accomplishments?
- What type of career (or work) excites you?
- What type of career (or work) is off-putting?

Power and Influence:

- What sets you apart from other leaders?
- What do you hope to gain from vetting the new initiative?
- Who do you need to influence?
- What behaviors/attitudes can you model that would gain the attention of your team?
- How will you begin the conversation with your stakeholders/team?
- What things are in your control that can be offered to your stakeholders/team?
- Who can you work with to help mobilize the stakeholders/team?

Leadership Presence (Human Capital and Leadership Behaviors):

- What are you values?
    - Which of these values are nonnegotiable?
- What is your vision?
- What are your strengths?
- Where can you improve?
- What is your idea of leadership growth and development?
    - How are you doing with this growth and development?
- How does your team view your leadership?
- What do you think is missing?
- How do you celebrate success with your team?
- What doubts do you have about your leadership abilities?
- How does your team view your communication abilities?

- How well do you engage and mobilize your team?
- How do you manage interruptions or disruptive behaviors?
- How do you ensure that your body language, tone, and behavior convey both authority and approachability?
- How do you influence others to adopt new ideas, strategies, or change initiatives?
- How do you plan to build and sustain your influence in the long term?
- What relationships or networks do you need to cultivate to enhance your future leadership power?
- How do you maintain a balance between assertiveness and humility when exercising influence?
- How can you demonstrate quick wins and early successes to build influence in a new setting?
- How do you help others in your team or organization build their own influence?
- How do you mentor emerging leaders to develop power and leadership presence?
- What role do you play in cultivating a culture of influence and empowerment within your team?

Stronger Teams:

- What is the goal/objective of the team?
- What roles/responsibilities are required of team members to achieve the goal?
- How can you (or the team leader) ensure that the team understands the expectations?
- What actions are in place to build team chemistry?
- What is/are each member's drivers?
- How can you (or the team leader) ensure that communication is open, honest, and transparent?
- How can you (or the team leader) establish trust?
- What procedures are in place to ensure that each team member is receiving feedback?
- How do you (or the team leader) display the following:
    - Empathy?
    - Social awareness?
    - Compassion?
    - Relationship management?

Communication:

- How would you describe your current communication style?
- What are the most common challenges you face when communicating with others?

- How does your team perceive your communication style?
- What aspects of your communication do you think are most effective?
- In what situations do you feel least confident about your communication skills?
- How do you ensure your message is clearly understood by others?
- When delivering a message, how do you gauge if the other person has understood you correctly?
- What techniques do you use to adjust your message based on your audience?
- How often do you find yourself fully listening versus thinking of your response during conversations?
- How can you demonstrate active listening in your conversations?
- What signals do you give to show others that you are truly listening to them?
- How do you manage your emotions when communicating in stressful situations?
- How aware are you of your body language and nonverbal cues when communicating?
- How can you ensure that your nonverbal communication aligns with what you're saying?
- What specific communication skills do you believe need improved?

Conflict Resolution/Negotiation:

- What strategies do you utilize when handling disagreement/conflict?
- What strategies do you use to manage or mitigate emotionally charged situations?
- What do you do to create a sense of trust amongst your team?
- How would you describe your current approach to negotiation?
- What do you think your strengths and weaknesses are when negotiating or resolving conflicts?
- How do you typically feel when faced with conflict or negotiation?
- How do you balance advocating for your own interests while understanding the needs of the other party?
- How do you manage your emotions when a negotiation becomes tense?
- How comfortable are you with exploring win–win solutions, where both parties can benefit?
- What strategies do you use to overcome deadlocks in negotiations?
- How do you handle situations where you feel your boundaries are being pushed or ignored?
- What specific negotiation skills would you like to improve?
- How will enhancing your conflict resolution abilities impact your career trajectory?

Some additional example questions from University of North Texas (n.d.) can be found here:

https://www.unthsc.edu/culture-and-experience/wp-content/uploads/sites/57/Powerful-Coaching-Questions_-brand.pdf

**Some questions in the list were generated using Chat GPT.*

Sites with Online Resources

As with textbooks, numerous online sites are available to provide useful tools and resources for coaches. Some are free, and some require a membership (paid or free). The following sites are provided as a launching pad to help the leader–coach find easy-to-use tools:

https://www.mindfulcoachingtools.com/free-tools

https://www.coachingtoolsshop.com/shop/all/free

https://www.thecoachingtoolscompany.com/free_coaching_tools/

https://www.mindtools.com/worksheets/Personal_SWOT_Analysis_Worksheet.pdf

Use of AI and Machine Learning

A resource section would not be complete without mention of AI. AI is now at the fingertips of every individual who has access to the internet or a smartphone. AI can help individuals and businesses alike to predict outcomes, generate recommendations, create text-based summaries, one-page papers, newsletters, blogs, activity sheets, and financial models, among other tasks—all in real time. This real-time, well-written output (with particular emphasis on ChatGPT) can be attractive and a go-to for busy professionals, but it should be utilized responsibly. At present, ChatGPT's output is only yielding about a 40% accuracy rate (Lopez, 2023). Thus, it should not be used to produce final products of any sort. Rather, users should use ChatGPT and other AI models as a launching pad for idea generation. Users should cross-reference content, use supporting literature and citations as appropriate, and acknowledge use of AI-generated content.

Reference

Lopez, J. (2023, August 13). *OpenAI's ChatGPT fools a third of users despite 52% wrong answers, Purdue study finds*. Tech Times. https://www.techtimes.com/articles/295041/20230813/openais-chatgpt-fools-third-users-despite-52-wrong-answers-purdue.htm

INDEX

A

accountability, 26, 97
ACHIEVE model of coaching, 119–120
Action Centered Leadership™, 31–32
active inquiry, 7–8, 25–26, 34, 43
active listening, 130–131
Adair, John, 31
adaptability, 116
adult learning theory, 3
'aha' moments, 8
Alderfer's ERG theory, 5
Alexander, Graham, 29
American Academy of Family Physicians (AAFP), 144–145
American Organization for Nursing Leadership (AONL), 43
ancillary service teams, 56
appreciative leadership, 145–146
artificial intelligence (AI), 66, 165
Association for Talent Development (ATD), 12
attribution feedback, 65
authentic leadership, 62, 106–107
  balanced processing, 101–102
  moral perspective, 102
  relational transparency, 101
  relationship between positive PsyCap and, 101
  self-awareness dimensions, 101
Authentic Leadership: Rediscovering the Secrets to Creating Lasting Value, 100
Authentic Leadership Questionnaire (ALQ), 107
Avolio, Bruce, 100

B

Bass, Bernard, 97
behavioral coaching, 51–53
  creating new behavior or response, 53
  identifying a behavior, 53
behavioral learning, 3–4
behaviorism, assumptions or principles of, 3
behavioristic psychology, 6
best alternative to a negotiated agreement (BATNA), 144–145
books, 153–155
Brown, Michael, 101
Burns, James McGregor, 96–97
buttering up concept, 50

C

career coaching, 43
career mentoring, 12
CEDAR feedback model, 68
changeology, 4
chaos theory, 5–6
charismatic leaders, 97
ChatGPT, 62, 66, 165
Clear Coaching, 16
CLEAR model of coaching, 31, 120
CliftonStrengths assessments, 23
coachable clients, 8
coach–client relationship, 7
  display of empathy, 9
  establishing trust in, 9–10
  sense of possibility, 9
coaching
  as client-driven, personalized process, 7
  background and history, 2–10
  books, 153–155
  case examples, 71–72
  circumstances appropriate for, 71
  conversations, 64–65, 70, 72–73
  definitions, 1–2
  differences between consulting, 10–12
  effective, 8–10
  essential principles, 6–8
  for conflict resolution, 146–147
  goals and action plans, 8–9, 136–137
  ICF coaching program, 153
  internal and external resources, 7
  online resources, 164
  personal issues and challenges, 7
  real-world application, 74
  research about, 15–16
  role in nurse leader role, 69–71
  templates, 155–164

coaching culture
  high-performance, 57
  human capital and, 79–80
  requirements, 80–81
coaching mindset, 62–63
coaching models
  Action Centered Leadership™, 31–32
  CLEAR model, 31
  GROW model, 29–30
  HILDA model, 33
  LAEDAN model, 34
  OSKAR/OSCAR model, 30–31
  SCARF model, 32–33
  STEPPPA model, 32
coaching process
  barriers or challenges, 26
  case example, 38–39
  clarification on interpretation of results, 25
  closure/celebration, 26
  initial assessment, 23–25
  plan and agenda, 26–29, 35–37
  problem identification or opportunity of interest, 21–22
  results check-in and action planning, 26
Coaching Skills (Jenny Rogers), 33
coercive power, 46
communication, 127–130
  approaches to improve, 134–135
  coaching to foster simple, strong, 136–137
complex adaptive systems, 6
confidentiality, 7
conflict
  in academic setting, 149–150
  in clinical situation, 148–149
  interpersonal, 140
  intrapersonal, 140
  task, 140
conflict resolution
  coaching for, 146–147
  five modes of, 141–142
  skills for, 116, 142–146
constructive development, 4
constructive feedback, 66
consulting
  as professional service, 10
  differences between coaching and, 10–12
  hierarchy of, 11
contingency feedback, 65
contingency teams, 55
continuous feedback, 66
coordinating teams, 55
core teams, 55
counseling, 13–14
  in multiple stages, 14
counterproductive work behaviors (CWB), 84
5C's model of high-performing teams, 116–117

D

360-degree assessments, 53
360-Degree feedback, 66
directive feedback, 65
DISC® personality assessment, 23–24
distance mentoring, 13
diversity-focused mentoring programs, 13

E

efficacy, 83
emotional intelligence, 15, 131–134, 144
  Goleman's model of, 131–132
  self-assessment, 132–134
"Emotionally Intelligent Leadership," 25
ethical standards, 7
evidence-based practice quality improvement (EBPQI), 119
executive coaching, 41–43
experience, role in adult learning, 3
expert nursing theory, 46
expert power, 45–46

F

feedback, 65
  feedback type or categorization and feedback delivery, 65–68
  formal, 65–66
  formative, 65–66
  impact, 65
  informal, 65–66
  loop, 137
  negative, 66
  peer, 136–137
  positive, 66
  summative, 65–66
  verbal, 66
  written, 66
financial capital, 77
Fine, Alan, 29
forethought, 83
formal 360 assessments, 23
formal feedback, 65–66
formal mentoring, 12

formative feedback, 65–66
The Future of Nursing 2020–2030: Charting a Path to Achieve Health Equity, 89

G

Generation Y and Generation Z—groups, 61–62, 69
Genos Emotional Intelligence assessment, 23–25
George, Bill, 100
Gilbert, Andrew, 30
Global Institute of Organizational Coaching, 2
Goleman's model of emotional intelligence, 131–132
group coaching, 137
group mentoring, 13
GROW model of coaching, 29–30, 119
GROW/RE-GROW framework, 85

H

habits, experimenting with and practicing, 5
hard tactics, 48
  coalition, 50
  ingratiation, 50
  legitimation, 49–50
  personal appeals, 50
  pressure tactics, 50
Hawkins, Peter, 31, 116–117
healthcare systems, 6
Hersey-Blanchard situational leadership model. *See* situational leadership
Herzberg's two-factor theory, 5
high-performing cultures, 57
high performing teams, 114–117
  5C's model of, 116–117
  adaptability, 116
  case examples, 123–124
  coaching to build, 118–119
  conflict resolution skills, 116
  culture of psychological safety, 118
  idea of creating or sustaining, 118
  leadership intervention and, 118
  professional and organizational outcomes, 117–118
  sense of accomplishment, 118
  trust, 114–116
  types of, 118–119
high potential employee mentoring, 13
HILDA model, 33
Hogan Assessments, 23–24
human capital, 78–79
  coaching culture and, 79–80
humanistic psychology, 6
humanistic theory, 4

I

ICF certified coaches, 62
ICF coaching program, 153
ideal self, 5
illumination, 145
impact feedback, 65
impulsive mind, 4
inclusion, 2, 89, 115, 117, 145–146
individual development, 31–32
informal feedback, 65–66
informal mentoring, 12
informational power, 47
inquiry, 58, 67, 145
  active, 7–8, 25–26, 34, 43
  topic of, 41–42
inspirational motivation, 97, 146
instrumental mind, 4
integral psychology, 6
integrity, 45, 99–102, 145–146
intellectual capital, 77–78
intellectual stimulation, 97–98
intended change theory, 5
interdisciplinary team collaboration, 121
interpersonal conflict, 140
interprofessional collaboration, 113–114
The Interprofessional Education Collaborative (IPEC), 113–114
intrapersonal conflict, 140
intrinsic motivation, 3

J

Jackson, Paul, 30
John Norcross's transtheoretical model of change, 4

K

Kegan, Robert, 4
knowledge-sharing mentoring, 13

L

LAEDAN model, 34
leadership. *See also* authentic leadership; situational leadership; transformational leadership
  assessments, 107–108
  growth and development, 41
  trust inside and outside the team, 114–115
Leadership Circle Profile (LCP), 23–24, 108

leadership coaching, 41–43
influencing behaviors, 47–51
need for shift in, 61–68
power use in, 44–47, 51
Leadership Practices Inventory (LPI), 108
learners' knowledge, role in adult learning, 3
learning agenda, 5
learning climate, 88
legitimate power, 44–45
listening, 8
active, 130–131

M

Management of Organizational Behavior: Utilizing Human Resources (Hersey-Blanchard), 103
Manchester Inc., 16
Maslow's hierarchy of needs, 4–5
McKergow, Mark, 30
McLeod, Angus, 32
mentoring, 11–13
MLQ + ALQ, 107
Multifactor Leadership Questionnaire (MLQ), 107
Myers-Briggs Type Indicator® (MBTI®), 23, 25

N

negative bargaining zone, 144
negative feedback, 66
new manager mentoring, 12
Noom program, 53
Northouse, Peter, 100
nursing burnout, 84
nursing team development, 122

O

observation, 83
one-one mentoring, 13
online resources, 164
open-ended questions, 8
optimism, 83–84
organizational behavior, 6, 57, 81–82
organizational citizenship behaviors (OCB), 84
organizational support, 88
orientation to learning, 3
OSKAR/OSCAR model, 30–31
OSKAR solution-focused model of coaching, 120–121

P

patient-centered care teams, 122–123
Pavlov, Ivan, 3
peer feedback, 136–137
peer mentoring, 13
performance coaching, 121. *See also* high performing teams
personal power, 47
personal relationships, 5
physical capital, 77
planning, 144
positive bargaining zone, 144
positive feedback, 66
positive organizational behavior or (POB), 82
positive organizational scholarship (POS), 82
positive psychology, 82, 86
post-coaching assessment, 56
powerful questions, 8
psychoanalytic psychology, 6
psychological capital, 78, 81–84
development and coaching, 84–87, 90
efficacy, 83
for nursing and nursing leadership development, 87–89
higher, 84
optimism, 83–84
resiliency, 83
workplace behaviors, 84

R

Raso, Rosanne, 101
readiness to learn, 3
real self, 5
referent power, 45
reflective practice, 137
relationship management, 132–133
resiliency, 83
return on investment (ROI), 16
reverse mentoring, 13
reward power, 44
Rogers, Carl, 4

S

SCARF model, 32–33
Schein's change theory, 5
self-actualization, 4
self-assessments, 136
self-authoring mind, 4
self-awareness, 24, 45, 51, 83, 100–101, 106, 131, 146–147
self-directedness, role in adult learning, 3
self-leadership development, 87–88
self-management, 24, 131
self-reflection, 83, 87, 137, 144–145, 148

self-regulation, 83
self-transforming mind, 4
Seligman, Dr. Martin, 81
situational leadership
  competencies, 103–105
  role of coaching, 105
  styles, 103
situation—behavior—impact (SBI) model for feedback, 67
SMART goal framework, 32, 86, 90, 114, 116, 136
Snyder's theory of hope, 82
social awareness, 132–133
social capital, 77
socialized mind, 4
social support, 88
soft tactics, 48–49
  appraising, 49
  collaboration, 49
  consultation, 49
  exchange, 48
  inspirational appeals, 49
  rational persuasion, 48
speed mentoring, 13
STEPPPA model, 32
stop—keep doing—start (SKS) feedback model, 68
strategic planning coaching, 54–55
strategy, 144–145
  implementation, 55
strengths, weaknesses, opportunities, and threats (SWOT) analysis, 54
summative feedback, 65–66
support services and administration teams, 56
symbolizing, 83

T

task achievement, 31
task conflict, 140
teaching, 15
team coaching, 55–56, 118–119
  considerations, 56
team information and management, 31
teams in healthcare, 55–56
teamwork, 113–117
technology-based learners, 61
templates, 155–164
Tracey, Bruce, 48
transformational leadership, 62, 95–96, 106–107
  background, 96–98
  building, 98–100
  embracing challenges, 99
  enabling others, 99–100
  idealized influence or charisma, 97
  individualized consideration, 98
  inspirational motivation, 97
  intellectual stimulation, 97–98
  recognition and celebrating contributions of others, 100
  shared vision, 99
transformational learning, 3
transpersonal psychology, 6

V

value creation, 144–145
verbal 360 assessments, 23
verbal feedback, 66
virtual team members, 119
Vroom's expectancy theory, 5

W

Watson, John B., 3
Wheatley, Margaret, 5
Whitmore, Sir John, 29
Whittleworth, Karen, 30
workplace behaviors, 84
written feedback, 66

Y

Yukl, Gary, 48

Z

zone of possible agreement (ZOPA), 144

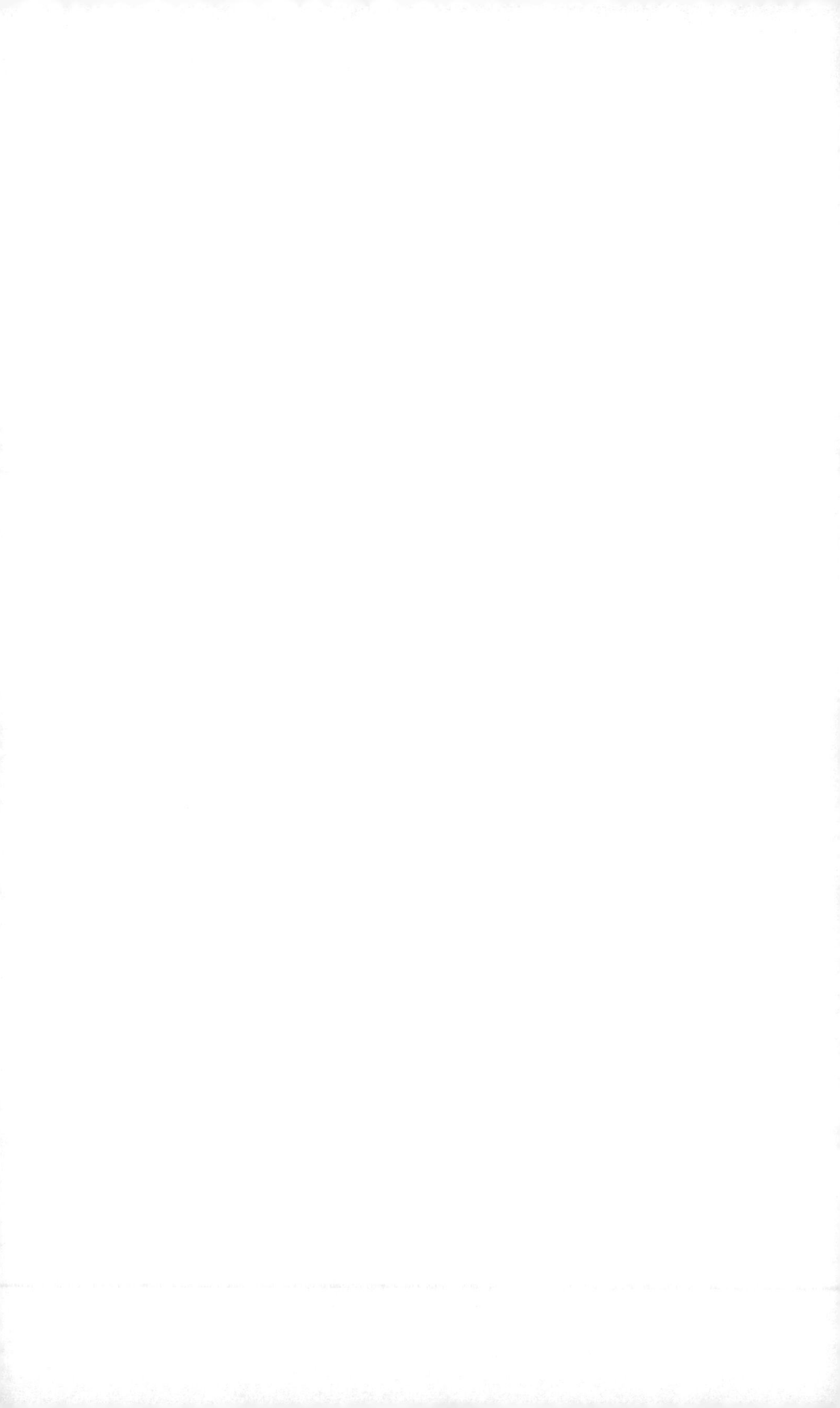

www.ingramcontent.com/pod-product-compliance
Ingram Content Group UK Ltd.
Pitfield, Milton Keynes, MK11 3LW, UK
UKHW021830270726
14058UKWH00001B/75

9 798823 338004